DIABETES DIETS AND RECIPES COOKBOOK

A Healthy Cookbook for Diabetes

D1716177

Dr Amber Richardson

TABLE OF CONTENT

INTRODUCTION

In the realm of health and wellness, few conditions demand as much attention and diligence as diabetes. From carefully monitoring blood sugar levels to making mindful dietary choices, managing diabetes requires a multifaceted approach. It's a journey filled with challenges, but also opportunities for empowerment and transformation.

Welcome to the "Diabetes Diets and Recipes Cookbook" – your trusted companion on this journey towards better health and vitality. Within the pages of this comprehensive guide, you'll find a wealth of knowledge, practical tips, and, most importantly, an array of delicious recipes specially crafted to support your diabetic lifestyle.

This cookbook is more than just a collection of recipes; it's a holistic resource designed to help you navigate the complexities of diabetes management with confidence and ease. Whether you're newly diagnosed, a seasoned veteran, or simply seeking fresh inspiration, you'll discover everything you need to thrive in your journey towards optimal health.

From hearty breakfasts to satisfying dinners, each recipe in this cookbook is thoughtfully curated to strike the perfect balance between flavor and nutrition. You'll find a variety of options to suit every taste preference and dietary need, ensuring that eating well never feels like a sacrifice.

But this book is about more than just what you put on your plate – it's about embracing a lifestyle that nurtures both body and soul. Throughout these pages, you'll find valuable insights into the science behind diabetes, practical tips for meal planning and preparation, and guidance on making sustainable lifestyle changes that promote long-term health and wellness.

Whether you're looking to manage your blood sugar levels, lose weight, or simply adopt a healthier way of eating, the "Diabetes Diets and Recipes Cookbook" is your ultimate resource for success. Let's embark on this journey together, one delicious meal at a time.

CHAPTER 1: Understanding Diabetes

What is Diabetes

Diabetes is a persistent health condition that disrupts the body's natural regulation of blood sugar, also known as glucose. Glucose is the primary source of energy for your cells, and its levels in your bloodstream are tightly regulated by the hormone insulin, which is produced by the pancreas. However, in people with diabetes, this delicate balance is disrupted, leading to elevated blood sugar levels that can have serious consequences if left unmanaged.

There are several types of diabetes, with the most common being type 1 and type 2 diabetes, as well as gestational diabetes which occurs during pregnancy.

Type 1 diabetes is an autoimmune condition in which the immune system mistakenly attacks and destroys the insulin-producing cells in the pancreas. This leads to insufficient insulin production, causing an elevation in blood sugar levels. Type 1 diabetes commonly emerges during childhood or adolescence, although it can manifest at any stage of life.

On the other hand, type 2 diabetes is characterized by insulin resistance, where the body's cells become resistant to the effects of insulin, and the pancreas is unable to produce enough insulin to compensate. This leads to elevated blood sugar levels. Type 2 diabetes is often associated with lifestyle factors such as obesity, physical inactivity, and poor diet, although genetics also play a significant role.

Gestational diabetes develops during pregnancy and is caused by hormonal changes that affect insulin sensitivity. While gestational diabetes usually resolves after childbirth, women who have had gestational diabetes are at increased risk of developing type 2 diabetes later in life.

Regardless of the type, diabetes can have serious consequences if left untreated or poorly managed. Chronic high blood sugar levels can damage blood vessels and nerves, leading to a variety of complications, including heart disease, stroke, kidney disease, vision problems, and nerve damage.

Managing diabetes requires a comprehensive approach that includes regular monitoring of blood sugar levels, adopting a healthy lifestyle, and, in some cases, taking medication or insulin injections. Diet plays a crucial role in diabetes management, as certain foods can cause blood sugar levels to spike while others help keep them stable.

A well-balanced diet for diabetes typically includes a variety of fruits, vegetables, whole grains, lean proteins, and healthy fats. Foods that are high in fiber, such as fruits, vegetables, and whole grains, are especially beneficial as they help slow down the absorption of glucose and prevent sharp spikes in blood sugar levels. Additionally, limiting the intake of sugary foods and refined carbohydrates can help keep blood sugar levels under control.

Physical activity is also an essential component of diabetes management, as it helps improve insulin sensitivity and promotes weight loss. Aim for at least 150 minutes of moderate-intensity exercise per week, such as brisk walking, swimming, or cycling, and incorporate strength training exercises at least twice a week to build muscle mass and improve overall health.

In addition to diet and exercise, medication or insulin therapy may be necessary to help control blood sugar levels in some cases. It's important to work closely with your healthcare team to develop a personalized treatment plan that meets your individual needs and goals.

By taking a proactive approach to managing diabetes through lifestyle changes, medication, and regular monitoring, you can minimize the risk of complications and lead a full and active life. With the right knowledge and support, living well with diabetes is not only possible but entirely achievable.

Importance of a Healthy Diet

A healthy diet is foundational to overall well-being and is instrumental in maintaining optimal health throughout life. It encompasses a balanced intake of various nutrients, including vitamins, minerals, proteins, carbohydrates, and fats, all of which are essential for the body's proper functioning. The significance of a healthy diet extends far beyond just providing nourishment; it plays a crucial role in disease prevention, energy production, cognitive function, and longevity.

One of the primary benefits of a healthy diet is its ability to prevent chronic diseases. Numerous studies have demonstrated the link between poor dietary habits and the development of conditions such as obesity, type 2 diabetes, heart disease, hypertension, and certain types of cancer. By adopting a diet rich in fruits, vegetables, whole grains, lean proteins, and healthy fats, individuals can significantly reduce their risk of developing these debilitating diseases. These foods are not only nutrient-dense but also contain phytochemicals and antioxidants that help protect the body against cellular damage and inflammation, two key factors in disease progression.

Furthermore, a healthy diet is essential for maintaining a healthy weight. Excess weight and obesity are significant risk factors for numerous health problems, including cardiovascular disease, diabetes, joint pain, and sleep apnea. By consuming a diet that is low in processed foods, added sugars, and unhealthy fats, individuals can more easily manage their weight and promote a healthier body composition. Additionally, incorporating regular physical activity into one's routine further enhances the benefits of a healthy diet by increasing energy expenditure and improving metabolic function.

Beyond physical health, a nutritious diet also plays a vital role in supporting cognitive function and mental well-being. Research has shown that certain nutrients, such as omega-3 fatty acids, antioxidants, and vitamins B6 and B12, are particularly important for brain health and may help reduce the risk of cognitive decline and neurodegenerative diseases like Alzheimer's. Furthermore, a diet rich in whole foods, such as fruits, vegetables, and whole grains, has been associated with a lower risk of depression and anxiety, as these foods provide essential nutrients that support neurotransmitter function and mood regulation.

In addition to preventing disease and promoting mental health, a healthy diet is crucial for sustaining energy levels and optimizing performance. Food is the body's primary source of fuel, and the types of foods consumed directly impact energy levels, concentration, and productivity. By choosing nutrient-dense foods that provide a steady supply of energy, individuals can avoid energy crashes and maintain peak performance throughout the day. Incorporating a balance of carbohydrates, proteins, and healthy fats into meals and snacks helps stabilize blood sugar levels and provides sustained energy to fuel both physical and mental activities. Furthermore, a healthy diet is essential for supporting optimal immune function. The immune system relies on a variety of nutrients, including vitamins A, C, D, and E, as well as zinc, selenium, and omega-3 fatty acids, to function properly. These nutrients help regulate immune responses, support the production of immune cells, and enhance the body's ability to fight off infections and diseases. By consuming a diet rich in fruits, vegetables, lean proteins, and whole grains, individuals can strengthen their immune system and reduce their susceptibility to illnesses.

The importance of a healthy diet cannot be overstated. It serves as the foundation for overall health and well-being, influencing everything from disease prevention and weight management to cognitive function and immune health. By prioritizing nutrient-rich foods and making mindful dietary choices, individuals can optimize their health and vitality, leading to a higher quality of life and a reduced risk of chronic diseases.

Benefits of Following a Diabetes Diet

A diabetes diet is not just a set of guidelines; it's a proactive approach to managing blood sugar levels and promoting overall health and well-being. By making mindful food choices and adhering to a balanced meal plan, individuals with diabetes can experience a multitude of benefits that extend beyond mere glucose control. Here are some comprehensive insights into the advantages of following a diabetes diet:

1. Blood Sugar Management: The primary goal of a diabetes diet is to regulate blood sugar levels to prevent spikes and crashes. By focusing on nutrient-dense foods with a low glycemic index, such as fruits, vegetables, whole grains, and lean proteins, individuals can maintain stable blood sugar levels throughout the day, reducing the risk of hyperglycemia and hypoglycemia.

2. Weight Management: Many individuals with diabetes struggle with weight management due to insulin resistance or medication side effects. A diabetes diet emphasizes portion control, calorie moderation, and balanced macronutrient intake, making it easier to achieve and maintain a healthy weight. By incorporating plenty of fiber-rich foods and lean proteins, individuals can feel full and satisfied while still controlling calorie intake.

3. Heart Health: Diabetes significantly increases the risk of cardiovascular disease, including heart attacks and strokes. However, a diabetes diet that is low in saturated fats, trans fats, cholesterol, and sodium can help reduce this risk by promoting heart-healthy eating habits. By choosing foods rich in omega-3 fatty acids, soluble fiber, and antioxidants, individuals can lower cholesterol levels, improve blood pressure, and support overall cardiovascular health.

4. Improved Energy Levels: Fluctuating blood sugar levels can lead to feelings of fatigue and lethargy in individuals with diabetes. By following a diabetes diet that focuses on slow-digesting carbohydrates, balanced meals, and regular eating patterns, individuals can stabilize their energy levels and avoid the energy crashes associated with rapid blood sugar fluctuations. Incorporating protein-rich snacks and staying hydrated can also help maintain energy throughout the day.

5. Prevention of Diabetes Complications: Uncontrolled diabetes can lead to serious complications such as nerve damage, kidney disease, vision problems, and circulation issues. However, by managing blood sugar levels through diet, individuals can significantly reduce the risk of developing these complications. A diabetes diet that prioritizes whole, nutrient-rich foods and limits processed sugars and refined carbohydrates can help protect against long-term complications and promote overall health.

6. Improved Insulin Sensitivity: Following a diabetes diet that focuses on whole foods, lean proteins, and healthy fats can improve insulin sensitivity, allowing cells to better respond to insulin and regulate blood sugar levels more effectively. This can reduce the need for insulin injections or other diabetes medications and may even lead to partial or complete remission of type 2 diabetes in some cases.

7. Enhanced Quality of Life: By following a diabetes diet and adopting healthy lifestyle habits, individuals can enjoy an improved quality of life with fewer diabetes-related symptoms and complications. Maintaining stable blood sugar levels, managing weight, and supporting overall health can lead to increased energy, better mood, and a greater sense of well-being.

Following a diabetes diet offers a multitude of benefits for individuals with diabetes, ranging from improved blood sugar management and weight control to reduced risk of complications and enhanced overall health and well-being. By making informed dietary choices and prioritizing nutrient-rich foods, individuals can take control of their diabetes management and lead healthier, happier lives.

CHAPTER 2: Planning a Diabetes Diet

Consulting with a Dietitian:

Navigating the complex landscape of nutrition and dietary choices can be challenging, especially for individuals with specific health concerns or goals. That's where the expertise of a registered dietitian (RD) or nutritionist becomes invaluable. Consulting with a dietitian offers personalized guidance, evidence-based recommendations, and ongoing support to help individuals achieve their health and wellness objectives. Here's a comprehensive look at the benefits and process of consulting with a dietitian:

1. Personalized Nutrition Assessment: One of the primary advantages of consulting with a dietitian is receiving a personalized nutrition assessment. Dietitians are trained to evaluate individuals' dietary habits, medical history, lifestyle factors, and health goals to develop tailored nutrition plans that meet their unique needs. This assessment may include a review of current eating patterns, nutrient intake, food preferences, allergies or intolerances, and any existing medical conditions or medications.

2. Goal Setting and Action Planning: Based on the nutrition assessment, a dietitian works collaboratively with clients to set realistic and achievable goals for improving their health and well-being. Whether the goal is weight management, blood sugar control, heart health, sports performance, or overall wellness, the dietitian helps clients identify specific objectives and develop actionable strategies to reach them. This may involve making dietary modifications, establishing meal plans, incorporating physical activity, and adopting behavior change techniques.

3. Evidence-Based Recommendations: Dietitians are trained in the latest scientific research and evidence-based practices in nutrition and dietetics. They provide accurate and up-to-date information on a wide range of nutrition topics, including macronutrients, micronutrients, dietary supplements, food allergies, and intolerances, as well as specialized diets for medical conditions such as diabetes, heart disease, gastrointestinal disorders, and autoimmune diseases. By staying informed about the latest research findings and guidelines, dietitians ensure that their recommendations are grounded in scientific evidence and best practices.

4. Nutrition Education and Counseling: In addition to providing recommendations, dietitians offer nutrition education and counseling to empower clients with the knowledge and skills they need to make informed dietary choices. This may involve teaching clients about the importance of balanced nutrition, portion control, meal planning, label reading, cooking techniques, and mindful eating practices. By understanding the fundamentals of nutrition, clients can make confident decisions about their diet and lifestyle to support their health goals.

5. Support and Accountability: Consulting with a dietitian provides ongoing support and accountability throughout the journey towards improved health and wellness. Dietitians serve as coaches and mentors, offering encouragement, motivation, and practical strategies to help clients overcome challenges and stay on track with their nutrition goals. Regular check-ins, follow-up appointments, and monitoring of progress allow dietitians to assess clients' progress, make adjustments to the nutrition plan as needed, and celebrate successes along the way.

6. Behavior Change Strategies: Changing dietary habits and adopting a healthier lifestyle can be challenging, but dietitians are equipped with behavioral change strategies to support clients in making lasting changes. They help clients identify barriers to change, develop coping strategies, set realistic expectations, and cultivate self-efficacy and confidence in their ability to achieve their goals. By addressing the psychological aspects of behavior change, dietitians empower clients to overcome obstacles and sustain positive dietary habits over the long term.

7. Collaboration with Healthcare Team: Dietitians often collaborate with other members of the healthcare team, including physicians, nurses, therapists, and other allied health professionals, to provide comprehensive care for clients. They may consult with healthcare providers to coordinate nutrition therapy with medical treatment plans, monitor progress, and address any nutrition-related concerns or complications. This interdisciplinary approach ensures that clients receive holistic care that addresses their unique health needs and goals.

Consulting with a dietitian offers numerous benefits for individuals seeking personalized nutrition guidance and support. From personalized nutrition assessments and evidence-based recommendations to nutrition education, counseling, and behavior change strategies, dietitians play a vital role in helping clients achieve their health and wellness goals. By working collaboratively with a dietitian, individuals can gain the knowledge, skills, and confidence they need to make sustainable dietary changes and optimize their health and well-being for the long term.

Setting Realistic Goals

Setting realistic goals is essential for achieving success in any endeavor, including health and wellness. Whether it's improving nutrition, increasing physical activity, or managing chronic conditions like diabetes, setting achievable goals helps individuals stay motivated, track progress, and maintain momentum towards their desired outcomes. Here's a comprehensive look at the importance of setting realistic goals and strategies for success:

1. Clarity and Focus: Setting specific, measurable, achievable, relevant, and time-bound (SMART) goals provides clarity and focus on what individuals want to accomplish. Instead of vague aspirations like "eat healthier" or "lose weight," setting specific goals such as "eat five servings of fruits and vegetables per day" or "lose 10 pounds in three months" provides a clear target to work towards. This clarity helps individuals prioritize their efforts and stay on track with their objectives.

2. Motivation and Commitment: Realistic goals provide motivation and commitment by giving individuals a sense of purpose and direction. When goals are attainable and within reach, individuals are more likely to stay motivated and committed to taking consistent action towards their goals. This sense of progress and achievement fuels momentum and encourages individuals to continue making positive changes in their behavior and lifestyle.

3. Progress Monitoring and Accountability: Setting realistic goals allows individuals to monitor their progress and hold themselves accountable for their actions. By breaking larger goals into smaller, manageable steps, individuals can track their achievements over time and celebrate milestones along the way. Regular progress monitoring provides valuable feedback on what's working well and where adjustments may be needed, helping individuals stay focused and motivated towards achieving their desired outcomes.

4. Adaptability and Flexibility: Realistic goals allow for adaptability and flexibility in the face of challenges or setbacks. Life is unpredictable, and obstacles are inevitable on the journey towards achieving goals. By setting realistic expectations and acknowledging that setbacks may occur, individuals can approach obstacles with resilience and creativity, finding alternative solutions and adjusting their goals as needed without becoming discouraged or giving up.

5. Risk Mitigation and Prevention of Burnout:
Setting realistic goals helps mitigate the risk of burnout and prevent feelings of overwhelm or frustration. Unrealistic goals that are too ambitious or aggressive can lead to disappointment and disillusionment if not achieved within a certain timeframe. By setting attainable goals that align with individuals' capabilities, resources, and constraints, individuals can avoid burnout and maintain a sustainable pace towards their goals.

6. Self-Efficacy and Confidence Building:
Achieving realistic goals builds self-efficacy and confidence, reinforcing individuals' belief in their ability to succeed. As individuals make progress towards their goals and overcome obstacles along the way, they develop a sense of competence and mastery that empowers them to

tackle new challenges with greater confidence and resilience. This positive feedback loop reinforces the belief that success is possible with effort and perseverance.

7. Long-Term Sustainability: Realistic goals promote long-term sustainability by focusing on gradual, sustainable changes that can be maintained over time. Crash diets, extreme exercise regimens, or rapid lifestyle changes may yield short-term results but are often unsustainable in the long run. By setting realistic goals that prioritize gradual progress and lifestyle modifications, individuals can establish habits that support their health and well-being for the long term.

Setting realistic goals is essential for achieving success in health and wellness endeavors. By providing clarity and focus, motivating commitment, facilitating progress monitoring and accountability, allowing for adaptability and flexibility, mitigating the risk of burnout, building self-efficacy and confidence, and promoting long-term sustainability, realistic goals empower individuals to make positive changes in their behavior and lifestyle that lead to lasting health and wellness outcomes. Whether it's improving nutrition, increasing physical activity, or managing chronic conditions, setting achievable goals lays the foundation for success and empowers individuals to live their best lives.

Creating a Meal Plan

A well-balanced meal plan is the cornerstone of a healthy lifestyle, providing the foundation for optimal nutrition, energy levels, and overall well-being. Whether the goal is to manage weight, support athletic performance, or address specific health concerns like diabetes or heart disease, creating a meal plan that is nutritious, balanced, and sustainable is essential. Here's a comprehensive guide to creating a meal plan that meets individual needs and goals:

1. Assessing Nutritional Needs: Before creating a meal plan, it's important to assess individual nutritional needs based on factors such as age, gender, weight, height, activity level, and health status. Consulting with a registered dietitian or nutritionist can provide personalized guidance and recommendations tailored to specific dietary requirements and goals. Additionally, considering cultural preferences, food allergies or intolerances, and budget constraints ensures that the meal plan is practical and realistic.

2. Setting Goals and Priorities: Determine the goals and priorities that will guide the meal planning process. Whether the goal is to lose weight, improve blood sugar control, increase energy levels, or support athletic performance, setting clear objectives helps focus efforts and tailor the meal plan accordingly. Prioritize nutrient-rich foods such as fruits, vegetables, whole grains, lean proteins, and healthy fats that provide essential vitamins, minerals, and antioxidants while minimizing added sugars, refined carbohydrates, and unhealthy fats.

3. Planning Meals and Snacks: Plan meals and snacks that provide a balance of macronutrients (carbohydrates, proteins, and fats) and micronutrients (vitamins and minerals) to meet nutritional needs throughout the day. Aim for three balanced meals and one to three nutrient-dense snacks, depending on individual preferences and energy requirements. Incorporate a variety of foods from all food groups to ensure a diverse and well-rounded diet that provides a wide range of nutrients.

4. Emphasizing Variety and Moderation:
Variety is key to a nutritious and enjoyable meal plan. Incorporate a diverse selection of foods from different food groups, including fruits, vegetables, whole grains, lean proteins, and healthy fats, to ensure adequate nutrient intake and prevent dietary boredom. Additionally, practice moderation when it comes to portion sizes and calorie intake to maintain a healthy weight and prevent overeating. Use portion control techniques such as measuring cups, food scales, or visual cues to ensure appropriate serving sizes.

5. Meal Prepping and Batch Cooking: Meal
prepping and batch cooking can save time and streamline the meal planning process by preparing ingredients or entire meals in advance. Choose one or two days per week to plan and prepare meals, portion out ingredients, and store them in convenient containers for easy access throughout the week. Batch cooking staples such

as grains, proteins, and vegetables allows for quick and convenient meal assembly, reducing the temptation to rely on unhealthy convenience foods or takeout meals.

6. Balancing Macronutrients: Balance meals and snacks with a combination of carbohydrates, proteins, and fats to support energy levels, satiety, and overall health. Choose complex carbohydrates such as whole grains, fruits, and vegetables, which provide fiber and slow-digesting carbohydrates that promote stable blood sugar levels and sustained energy. Include lean proteins such as poultry, fish, tofu, legumes, and dairy products to support muscle growth and repair, as well as healthy fats such as avocados, nuts, seeds, and olive oil, which provide essential fatty acids and promote heart health.

7. Listening to Hunger and Fullness Cues: Pay attention to hunger and fullness cues to guide meal timing and portion sizes. Eat when hungry and stop when satisfied, rather than relying on external cues such as meal times or portion sizes. Practice mindful eating by savoring each bite, chewing slowly, and paying attention to hunger and fullness signals to prevent overeating and promote a healthy relationship with food.

8. Staying Flexible and Adaptable: Flexibility and adaptability are key to maintaining a sustainable meal plan. Life is unpredictable, and there will inevitably be occasions when plans change or unexpected events occur. Instead of rigidly adhering to a strict meal plan, be flexible and willing to make adjustments as needed. Have a repertoire of quick and easy meal ideas, pantry staples, and go-to recipes for busy days or times when fresh ingredients are unavailable.

9. Seeking Support and Accountability: Seeking support and accountability from friends, family members, or a registered dietitian can help maintain motivation and adherence to the meal plan. Share goals and progress with others, join a support group or online community, or enlist the help of a dietitian for guidance, encouragement, and accountability. Having a support system in place can provide valuable feedback, encouragement, and motivation to stay on track with healthy eating habits.

10. Evaluating and Adjusting: Periodically evaluate the meal plan to assess progress, identify areas for improvement, and make necessary adjustments. Monitor weight, energy levels, hunger and fullness cues, blood sugar levels (if applicable), and overall well-being to gauge the effectiveness of the meal plan. Be open to feedback and willing to experiment with different foods, recipes, and meal timing strategies to optimize results and ensure long-term success.

Creating a meal plan is a proactive and empowering approach to achieving health and wellness goals. By assessing nutritional needs, setting realistic goals, planning balanced meals and snacks, emphasizing variety and moderation, practicing meal prepping and batch cooking, balancing macronutrients, listening to hunger and fullness cues, staying flexible and adaptable, seeking support and accountability, and evaluating and adjusting as needed, individuals can develop a sustainable meal plan that supports their health, energy levels, and overall well-being. With careful planning and mindful choices, creating and sticking to a nutritious meal plan can lay the foundation for a lifetime of health and vitality.

Monitoring Carbohydrate Intake

Monitoring carbohydrate intake is a fundamental aspect of managing various health conditions, including diabetes, obesity, and metabolic syndrome. Carbohydrates are the body's primary source of energy, but they can also have a significant impact on blood sugar levels, insulin sensitivity, and weight management. By monitoring carbohydrate intake and making informed dietary choices, individuals can better control blood sugar levels, optimize metabolic health, and achieve their health and wellness goals. Here's a comprehensive guide to monitoring carbohydrate intake:

1. Understanding Carbohydrates:
Carbohydrates are one of the three macronutrients found in food, along with protein and fat. They are classified into three main categories: sugars, starches, and fiber. Sugars are simple carbohydrates found naturally in fruits, vegetables, dairy products, and added sugars in processed foods. Starches, classified as complex

carbohydrates, are prevalent in grains, legumes, and starchy vegetables. Fiber is a type of carbohydrate found in plant-based foods that provides numerous health benefits, including improved digestion, satiety, and blood sugar control.

2. Assessing Carbohydrate Needs: The amount of carbohydrates needed varies depending on individual factors such as age, gender, weight, height, activity level, metabolic rate, and health status. Individuals with diabetes, for example, may need to monitor carbohydrate intake more closely to manage blood sugar levels effectively. Consulting with a registered dietitian or certified diabetes educator can provide personalized guidance on carbohydrate goals and meal planning strategies tailored to individual needs and preferences.

3. Counting Carbohydrates: Carbohydrate counting is a method used to track the grams of carbohydrates consumed at each meal and snack to help manage blood sugar levels. It involves reading food labels, estimating portion sizes, and keeping track of carbohydrate intake throughout the day. Carbohydrate counting can be done using various methods, including carbohydrate exchanges, grams of carbohydrate per serving, or glycemic index/load values. A dietitian can teach carbohydrate counting techniques and provide resources such as carbohydrate counting guides and meal planning tools to assist with tracking carbohydrate intake.

4. Choosing Carbohydrate Sources Wisely: Not all carbohydrates are created equal, and choosing carbohydrate sources wisely can have a significant impact on blood sugar levels, satiety, and overall health. Opt for nutrient-dense carbohydrates that are rich in fiber, vitamins, minerals, and antioxidants, such as fruits, vegetables, whole grains, legumes, and dairy products. These foods provide sustained energy, promote feelings of fullness, and support overall health and well-being. Limit or avoid refined carbohydrates, added sugars, and processed foods that provide empty calories and contribute to blood sugar spikes, weight gain, and chronic diseases.

5. Balancing Carbohydrates with Protein and Fat: Balancing carbohydrates with protein and fat helps stabilize blood sugar levels, promote satiety, and prevent energy crashes. Include lean proteins such as poultry, fish, tofu, legumes, and dairy products, as well as healthy fats such as avocados, nuts, seeds, and olive oil, in meals and snacks to slow down the absorption of carbohydrates and provide sustained energy. Aim for a balanced combination of carbohydrates, protein, and fat at each meal and snack to optimize metabolic health and support overall well-being.

6. Monitoring Blood Sugar Levels: Regular blood sugar monitoring is essential for assessing the impact of carbohydrate intake on blood sugar levels and making necessary adjustments to the meal plan. Testing before and after meals, as well as at various times throughout the day, can help identify patterns and trends and guide dietary modifications. It's important to work with a healthcare provider to establish target blood sugar ranges and develop an individualized monitoring plan.

7. Adjusting Carbohydrate Intake: Adjust carbohydrate intake based on individual responses to food, physical activity levels, medication regimen, and health goals.

Experiment with different carbohydrate sources, portion sizes, and meal timing strategies to find what works best for managing blood sugar levels and optimizing metabolic health. Be mindful of carbohydrate-rich foods that may cause blood sugar spikes and adjust intake accordingly. Consult with a registered dietitian or certified diabetes educator for personalized guidance on carbohydrate management and meal planning strategies.

8. Maintaining Consistency: Consistency in carbohydrate intake and meal timing is key for managing blood sugar levels and preventing fluctuations. Aim to eat meals and snacks at regular intervals throughout the day and avoid skipping meals or going long periods without eating. Consistent carbohydrate intake helps stabilize blood sugar levels, support energy levels, and prevent overeating or undereating.

9. Staying Informed and Educated: Stay informed about the latest research, guidelines, and recommendations related to carbohydrate intake and blood sugar management. Attend educational workshops, seminars, or support groups focused on diabetes management and nutrition. Keep up-to-date with reliable sources of information from reputable organizations such as the American Diabetes Association, Academy of Nutrition and Dietetics, and Centers for Disease Control and Prevention.

10. Seeking Support and Guidance: Managing carbohydrate intake and blood sugar levels can be challenging, but individuals don't have to do it alone. Seek support from healthcare providers, registered dietitians, certified diabetes educators, support groups, and online communities. These resources can provide valuable guidance, encouragement, and practical strategies for managing carbohydrate intake, optimizing metabolic health, and achieving long-term success in diabetes management.

Monitoring carbohydrate intake is an essential component of managing blood sugar levels, optimizing metabolic health, and achieving overall well-being. By understanding carbohydrates, assessing individual needs, counting carbohydrates, choosing carbohydrate sources wisely, balancing carbohydrates with protein and fat, monitoring blood sugar levels, adjusting carbohydrate intake as needed, maintaining consistency, staying informed and educated, and seeking support and guidance, individuals can effectively manage carbohydrate intake and achieve their health and wellness goals. With careful monitoring and informed dietary choices, individuals can empower themselves to take control of their health and live their best lives.

CHAPTER 3: Essential Nutrients for Diabetes

Carbohydrates and Blood Sugar

Carbohydrates are a macronutrient found in various foods and beverages, ranging from fruits and vegetables to grains and dairy products. When consumed, carbohydrates are broken down into glucose, the body's primary source of energy. Glucose is then absorbed into the bloodstream, where it circulates and provides fuel for cells throughout the body. However, the relationship between carbohydrates and blood sugar is complex, especially for individuals with diabetes or those seeking to manage their blood sugar levels. Here's a comprehensive guide to understanding carbohydrates and their impact on blood sugar:

1. Types of Carbohydrates: Carbohydrates are classified into three main types: sugars, starches, and fiber. Sugars, such as glucose, fructose, and sucrose, are simple carbohydrates found naturally in fruits, vegetables, and dairy products, as well as added sugars in processed foods and beverages. Complex carbohydrates known as starches are present in grains, legumes, and starchy vegetables such as potatoes and corn. Additionally, fiber, another type of carbohydrate, is abundant in plant-based foods like fruits, vegetables, whole grains, nuts, and seeds. Each type of carbohydrate has a different effect on blood sugar levels due to differences in their chemical structure and how they are digested and absorbed by the body.

2. Glycemic Index and Glycemic Load: The glycemic index (GI) is a measure of how quickly carbohydrates in a particular food raise blood sugar levels after consumption. Foods with a high GI, such as white bread, white rice, and sugary snacks, cause a rapid spike in blood sugar levels, followed by a rapid drop. In contrast, foods with a low GI, such as whole grains, fruits, and vegetables, cause a slower and more gradual rise in blood sugar levels. The glycemic load (GL) takes into account both the quantity and quality of carbohydrates in a serving of food, providing a more accurate measure of its impact on blood sugar levels.

3. Blood Sugar Regulation: The body has intricate mechanisms for regulating blood sugar levels and keeping them within a narrow range to ensure adequate energy supply for cells and tissues. When blood sugar levels rise after consuming carbohydrates, the pancreas releases insulin, a hormone that helps cells absorb glucose from the bloodstream and convert it into energy or store it for later use. In individuals with diabetes, this process is impaired, leading to elevated blood sugar levels and potential complications if left uncontrolled.

4. Impact of Carbohydrates on Blood Sugar: Carbohydrates have the most significant impact on blood sugar levels compared to other macronutrients like protein and fat. Simple carbohydrates, such as sugars and refined grains, are quickly digested and absorbed into the bloodstream, causing a rapid spike in blood sugar levels. Complex carbohydrates, such as whole grains, legumes, and fiber-rich foods, are digested more slowly, resulting in a gradual and sustained release of glucose into the bloodstream. This slower digestion and absorption help prevent sharp fluctuations in blood sugar levels and promote better overall blood sugar control.

5. Carbohydrate Counting: Carbohydrate counting is a common strategy used by individuals with diabetes to manage their blood sugar levels. It involves tracking the grams of carbohydrates consumed at each meal and snack and adjusting insulin doses or medication accordingly. Carbohydrate counting allows individuals to anticipate the impact of carbohydrate-containing foods on blood sugar levels and make informed dietary choices to support optimal blood sugar control. Working with a registered dietitian or certified diabetes educator can help individuals learn carbohydrate counting techniques and develop personalized meal plans tailored to their individual nutritional needs and health goals.

6. Role of Fiber: Fiber plays a crucial role in blood sugar regulation and overall health. Soluble fiber, found in foods like oats, legumes, fruits, and vegetables, helps slow down the absorption of glucose into the bloodstream, leading to more stable blood sugar levels. Insoluble fiber, found in foods like whole grains, nuts, and seeds, promotes digestive health and may also have beneficial effects on blood sugar control. Including fiber-rich foods in meals and snacks can help individuals with diabetes manage their blood sugar levels and support overall health and well-being.

7. Timing and Portion Control: The timing and portion sizes of carbohydrate-containing foods also play a role in blood sugar management. Eating carbohydrates in combination with protein, healthy fats, and fiber-rich foods can help slow down the absorption of glucose into the bloodstream and prevent sharp spikes in blood sugar levels. Additionally, spreading carbohydrate intake evenly throughout the day and controlling portion sizes can help prevent overeating and promote more stable blood sugar levels.

Carbohydrates play a significant role in blood sugar regulation, and understanding their impact is essential for individuals with diabetes or those seeking to manage their blood sugar levels effectively. By choosing carbohydrates wisely, monitoring portion sizes, practicing carbohydrate counting, including fiber-rich foods in meals and snacks, and paying attention to timing, individuals can support optimal blood sugar control and promote overall health and well-being. Working with a healthcare provider or registered dietitian can provide personalized guidance and support for managing carbohydrate intake and achieving blood sugar management goals.

Protein for Sustained Energy

Protein is an essential macronutrient that plays numerous critical roles in the body, including building and repairing tissues, supporting immune function, and serving as a source of energy. While carbohydrates are traditionally associated with providing energy, protein also plays a significant role in sustaining energy levels over the long term. Here's a comprehensive look at how protein contributes to sustained energy and why it's essential for overall health and well-being:

1. Slow and Sustained Release of Energy: Unlike carbohydrates, which are quickly broken down into glucose and rapidly absorbed into the bloodstream, protein is digested and metabolized at a slower pace. This slower digestion process results in a more gradual and sustained release of energy, helping to maintain stable blood sugar levels and prevent energy crashes throughout the day. Consuming protein-rich foods at meals and snacks can help provide a steady source of energy to fuel physical activity, cognitive function, and daily tasks.

2. Muscle Preservation and Repair: Protein is the building block of muscles, tissues, and organs in the body. Consuming an adequate amount of protein is essential for preserving lean muscle mass, supporting muscle repair and recovery, and optimizing physical performance. During periods of increased activity or exercise, the body relies on protein to repair damaged muscle fibers and build new muscle tissue, which contributes to overall strength, endurance, and energy levels.

3. Appetite Regulation and Satiety: Protein has been shown to have a significant impact on appetite regulation and feelings of fullness. Including protein-rich foods in meals and snacks can help increase satiety and reduce hunger, which may prevent overeating and promote weight management. Unlike carbohydrates, which can cause rapid fluctuations in blood sugar levels and lead to cravings and energy crashes, protein helps stabilize blood sugar levels and promote a more balanced and sustainable approach to eating.

4. Thermic Effect of Food (TEF): Protein has a higher thermic effect of food (TEF) compared to carbohydrates and fats, meaning that it requires more energy to digest, absorb, and metabolize. This increased metabolic rate following protein consumption contributes to greater calorie expenditure and may help support weight management efforts. By choosing protein-rich foods, individuals can increase their overall energy expenditure and promote fat loss while preserving lean muscle mass.

5. Nutrient Density and Micronutrients: Protein-rich foods are often nutrient-dense, meaning they provide a wide range of essential vitamins, minerals, and micronutrients in addition to protein. These micronutrients play crucial roles in energy metabolism, enzyme function, and overall health and well-being. Consuming a variety of protein sources, such as lean meats, poultry, fish, eggs, dairy products, legumes, nuts, and seeds, ensures adequate intake of essential nutrients that support energy production and vitality.

6. Blood Sugar Regulation: Protein can help stabilize blood sugar levels and prevent spikes and crashes that can lead to fluctuations in energy levels. When consumed with carbohydrates, protein slows down the absorption of glucose into the bloodstream, resulting in a more gradual rise and fall in blood sugar levels. This balanced approach to eating helps prevent energy dips and promotes sustained energy levels throughout the day.

7. Adaptability and Versatility: Protein is a versatile nutrient that can be incorporated into a wide range of meals and snacks to support sustained energy. Whether it's adding lean protein sources like chicken breast or tofu to salads, enjoying Greek yogurt or cottage cheese as a snack, or incorporating protein-rich smoothies or shakes into post-workout recovery, there are countless ways to include protein in the diet and optimize energy levels.

Protein plays a crucial role in providing sustained energy for physical activity, cognitive function, and daily tasks. By consuming protein-rich foods at meals and snacks, individuals can benefit from a slow and steady release of energy, improved appetite regulation and satiety, preservation of lean muscle mass, increased calorie expenditure, and enhanced nutrient density. Including a variety of protein sources in the diet ensures adequate intake of essential nutrients while supporting overall health and well-being. Whether it's lean meats, poultry, fish, eggs, dairy products, legumes, nuts, or seeds, prioritizing protein-rich foods is essential for sustaining energy levels and promoting optimal health and vitality.

Healthy Fats and Heart Health

Fats are an essential macronutrient that provides energy, supports cell growth, and helps the body absorb certain vitamins. While it's important to consume fats in moderation, not all fats are created equal. Healthy fats, also known as unsaturated fats, play a crucial role in promoting heart health and reducing the risk of cardiovascular disease. Here's a comprehensive look at the benefits of healthy fats for heart health and how to incorporate them into a balanced diet:

1. Types of Healthy Fats: Healthy fats are divided into two main categories: monounsaturated fats and polyunsaturated fats. Monounsaturated fats, found in foods like olive oil, avocado, and nuts, have been associated with lower levels of LDL (bad) cholesterol and reduced risk of heart disease. Polyunsaturated fats, including omega-3 and omega-6 fatty acids, are found in fatty fish (such as salmon, mackerel, and sardines), flaxseeds, chia seeds, walnuts, and soybean oil. Omega-3 fatty acids, in particular, have anti-inflammatory properties and are known for their heart-protective effects.

2. Cholesterol Management: Healthy fats can help improve cholesterol levels and reduce the risk of atherosclerosis, a condition characterized by the buildup of plaque in the arteries. Monounsaturated and polyunsaturated fats have been shown to lower LDL cholesterol levels while increasing HDL (good) cholesterol levels, leading to a more favorable lipid profile. By replacing saturated and trans fats with healthy fats in the diet, individuals can help manage cholesterol levels and reduce their risk of cardiovascular disease.

3. Inflammation Reduction: Chronic inflammation is a key driver of cardiovascular disease and other chronic conditions. Omega-3 fatty acids, found in fatty fish and plant-based sources like flaxseeds and walnuts, have potent anti-inflammatory properties that can help reduce inflammation in the body. By incorporating omega-3-rich foods into the diet, individuals can help mitigate inflammation and lower their risk of heart disease and other inflammatory conditions.

4. Blood Pressure Regulation: High blood pressure, or hypertension, is a significant risk factor for heart disease and stroke. Monounsaturated and polyunsaturated fats have been shown to help lower blood pressure levels and improve overall cardiovascular health. These fats can help relax blood vessels, improve blood flow, and reduce the workload on the heart, leading to better blood pressure control and reduced risk of hypertension-related complications.

5. Blood Sugar Management: Healthy fats can also play a role in blood sugar management and diabetes prevention. By slowing down the absorption of carbohydrates and preventing rapid spikes in blood sugar levels, healthy fats can help promote stable blood sugar control and reduce the risk of insulin resistance and type 2 diabetes. Including healthy fats in meals and snacks can help improve glycemic control and support overall metabolic health.

6. Antioxidant Absorption: Certain vitamins and antioxidants, such as vitamin E and carotenoids, are fat-soluble, meaning they need to be consumed with dietary fat to be properly absorbed and utilized by the body. Healthy fats help enhance the absorption of these nutrients, which have been linked to improved heart health and reduced risk of cardiovascular disease. Incorporating sources of healthy fats into meals rich in antioxidants, such as fruits, vegetables, and whole grains, can maximize their health benefits and support overall well-being.

7. Moderation and Balance: While healthy fats offer numerous health benefits, it's important to consume them in moderation as part of a balanced diet. Fats are calorie-dense, so portion control is key to maintaining a healthy weight and preventing excessive calorie intake. Aim to replace unhealthy fats, such as saturated fats and trans fats found in fried foods, processed snacks, and baked goods, with healthier alternatives like olive oil, avocado, nuts, seeds, and fatty fish.

Healthy fats play a crucial role in promoting heart health and reducing the risk of cardiovascular disease. By incorporating sources of monounsaturated and polyunsaturated fats into a balanced diet, individuals can help manage cholesterol levels, reduce inflammation, lower blood pressure, improve blood sugar control, enhance antioxidant absorption, and support overall cardiovascular health. Prioritizing foods like olive oil, avocado, nuts, seeds, fatty fish, and plant-based oils can contribute to better heart health and long-term well-being.

Importance of Fiber

Fiber is a type of carbohydrate found in plant-based foods that is essential for maintaining optimal health and well-being. Despite being classified as a carbohydrate, fiber is unique in that it cannot be fully digested or absorbed by the body. Instead, it moves through the digestive tract without being fully broken down or absorbed, offering a multitude of health advantages. From supporting digestive health to reducing the risk of chronic diseases, fiber plays a crucial role in overall health. Here's a comprehensive look at the importance of fiber and why it should be a staple in everyone's diet:

1. Digestive Health: One of the primary roles of fiber is to promote digestive health. Insoluble fiber, found in foods like whole grains, nuts, seeds, and the skin of fruits and vegetables, adds bulk to stool and helps prevent constipation by promoting regular bowel movements. Soluble fiber, found in foods like oats, legumes, fruits, and vegetables, forms a gel-like substance in the digestive tract, which helps soften stool and promote regularity. By supporting proper digestion and bowel function, fiber helps maintain a healthy digestive system and prevent digestive issues like constipation, diarrhea, and diverticulosis.

2. Weight Management: Fiber-rich foods are often lower in calories and higher in volume, which can help promote feelings of fullness and satiety. Including fiber-rich foods in meals and snacks can help reduce hunger and prevent overeating, making it easier to manage weight and prevent weight gain. Additionally, fiber helps slow down the digestion and absorption of carbohydrates, which can help stabilize blood sugar levels and prevent energy crashes that may lead to cravings and overeating. By promoting satiety and regulating appetite, fiber plays a role in supporting healthy weight management and preventing obesity.

3. Blood Sugar Control: Soluble fiber has been shown to help improve blood sugar control by slowing down the absorption of glucose into the bloodstream. This can help prevent rapid spikes in blood sugar levels after meals and promote more stable blood sugar levels throughout the day. By improving insulin sensitivity and reducing insulin resistance, fiber-rich foods may help reduce the risk of type 2 diabetes and improve glycemic control in individuals with diabetes. Including fiber-rich foods in meals and snacks can help support overall metabolic health and reduce the risk of chronic diseases associated with insulin resistance and elevated blood sugar levels.

4. Heart Health: Fiber has been linked to a reduced risk of heart disease and stroke due to its ability to lower cholesterol levels and improve other heart disease risk factors. Soluble fiber binds to cholesterol in the digestive tract and helps remove it from the body, leading to lower LDL (bad) cholesterol levels and a reduced risk of atherosclerosis. Additionally, fiber helps regulate blood pressure levels and reduce inflammation, both of which are important for maintaining cardiovascular health. Including fiber-rich foods like oats, barley, beans, lentils, fruits, and vegetables as part of a heart-healthy diet can help support overall cardiovascular health and reduce the risk of heart disease and stroke.

5. Gut Microbiota: Fiber serves as a prebiotic, which means it provides fuel for beneficial bacteria in the gut known as probiotics. These beneficial bacteria help maintain a healthy balance of microorganisms in the gut microbiota, which is essential for proper digestion, immune function, and overall health. By promoting the growth of beneficial bacteria, fiber helps support a healthy gut microbiome and may reduce the risk of digestive disorders, inflammatory bowel disease, and other gastrointestinal conditions.

Fiber is a crucial nutrient that plays a key role in supporting digestive health, weight management, blood sugar control, heart health, and gut microbiota. Including a variety of fiber-rich foods in the diet, such as whole grains, fruits, vegetables, legumes, nuts, and seeds, can help individuals reap the numerous health benefits associated with fiber. By prioritizing fiber-rich foods as part of a balanced diet, individuals can support overall health and well-being and reduce the risk of chronic diseases.

CHAPTER 4: Breakfast Recipes

High-Fiber Oatmeal

Oatmeal is a popular breakfast choice that offers a wide range of health benefits, especially when prepared with high-fiber ingredients. High-fiber oatmeal provides a satisfying and nutritious start to the day, offering a combination of soluble and insoluble fiber, vitamins, minerals, and antioxidants. Here's a comprehensive look at the benefits of high-fiber oatmeal and how to make it a delicious and nourishing breakfast option:

1. Heart Health: Oats are rich in soluble fiber, specifically a type called beta-glucan, which has been shown to help lower LDL (bad) cholesterol levels and reduce the risk of heart disease. Consuming high-fiber oatmeal regularly can help promote heart health by lowering cholesterol levels, improving blood vessel function, and reducing inflammation in the body.

2. Digestive Health: High-fiber oatmeal is beneficial for digestive health due to its high fiber content. The soluble fiber in oats helps soften stool and promote regular bowel movements, while the insoluble fiber adds bulk to stool and helps prevent constipation. Including high-fiber oatmeal in your diet can help support digestive regularity and prevent digestive issues like constipation and bloating.

3. Blood Sugar Control: Oats have a low glycemic index, meaning they cause a gradual and steady increase in blood sugar levels compared to refined carbohydrates. The soluble fiber in oats helps slow down the absorption of glucose into the bloodstream, which can help improve blood sugar control and reduce the risk of insulin resistance and type 2 diabetes. Consuming high-fiber oatmeal as part of a balanced breakfast can help stabilize blood sugar levels and provide sustained energy throughout the morning.

4. Weight Management: High-fiber oatmeal is a filling and satisfying breakfast option that can help promote weight management. The combination of soluble and insoluble fiber in oats helps increase feelings of fullness and satiety, which can reduce overall calorie intake and prevent overeating later in the day. Starting the day with a bowl of high-fiber oatmeal can help curb cravings, prevent snacking between meals, and support healthy weight loss or maintenance goals.

5. Versatility and Flavor: High-fiber oatmeal is incredibly versatile and can be customized with a variety of toppings and flavorings to suit individual preferences. Add-ins such as fresh or dried fruit, nuts, seeds, nut butter, spices, and sweeteners like honey or maple syrup can enhance the flavor and nutritional profile of oatmeal. Experiment with different combinations to create delicious and satisfying breakfast bowls that you'll look forward to enjoying each morning.

To make high-fiber oatmeal, start by cooking rolled or steel-cut oats according to package instructions. For added fiber and nutrition, consider stirring in ground flaxseeds, chia seeds, or wheat germ during cooking. Once cooked, top your oatmeal with a variety of high-fiber toppings such as berries, sliced bananas, chopped nuts, seeds, or a dollop of Greek yogurt. Drizzle with a touch of honey or maple syrup for sweetness if desired. Enjoy your high-fiber oatmeal warm and creamy for a nourishing and satisfying breakfast that will keep you fueled and energized throughout the morning.

Veggie Omelet

The veggie omelet is a versatile and nutrient-packed breakfast dish that combines eggs with a variety of vegetables for a satisfying and flavorful meal. Whether you're looking to add more vegetables to your diet, boost your protein intake, or simply enjoy a delicious and filling breakfast, the veggie omelet is a fantastic choice. Here's a comprehensive look at the benefits of the veggie omelet and how to make it a delicious and nutritious addition to your morning routine:

1. Nutrient-Rich Ingredients: The veggie omelet is packed with a wide range of nutrients from both the eggs and the vegetables. Eggs are an excellent source of high-quality protein, providing all nine essential amino acids that the body needs for muscle repair, growth, and maintenance. Additionally, eggs are rich in vitamins and minerals, including vitamin D, vitamin B12, selenium, and choline. By adding a variety of vegetables such as spinach, bell peppers, onions, mushrooms, tomatoes, and zucchini to the omelet, you can further boost its nutrient content with fiber, vitamins, minerals, and antioxidants.

2. Heart Health Benefits: The veggie omelet can be part of a heart-healthy diet due to its nutrient-rich ingredients and low saturated fat content. Eggs have been shown to have a neutral or positive effect on heart health when consumed as part of a balanced diet. Additionally, vegetables are low in calories and rich in fiber, which can help promote heart health by reducing cholesterol levels, improving blood pressure, and supporting overall cardiovascular function. By choosing heart-healthy cooking methods such as cooking with olive oil or avocado oil and limiting added salt and cheese, you can create a delicious and nutritious veggie omelet that supports heart health.

3. Weight Management: The veggie omelet is a satisfying and filling breakfast option that can help support weight management goals. Eggs are a nutrient-dense food that provides satiety and helps curb cravings, making them an excellent choice for those looking to control appetite and reduce calorie intake. Additionally, vegetables are low in calories and high in fiber, which adds bulk to the omelet without adding excess calories. By including plenty of vegetables in your veggie omelet, you can create a hearty and satisfying meal that keeps you feeling full and satisfied until your next meal.

4. Versatility and Customization: One of the best things about the veggie omelet is its versatility and customization options. You can customize your omelet with your favorite vegetables, herbs, spices, and cheeses to create a personalized breakfast masterpiece. Experiment with different combinations of vegetables to create unique flavor profiles and add variety to your breakfast routine. Whether you prefer a classic combination like spinach and feta or a more adventurous mix like mushrooms and goat cheese, the veggie omelet offers endless possibilities for delicious and nutritious breakfasts.

To make a veggie omelet, start by whisking eggs in a bowl and seasoning with salt, pepper, and any desired herbs or spices. Heat a non-stick skillet over medium heat and add a small amount of olive oil or cooking spray. Add your choice of chopped vegetables to the skillet and cook until softened. Pour the whisked eggs over the vegetables, tilting the skillet to spread the eggs evenly. Cook the omelet for a few minutes, gently lifting the edges with a spatula to allow the uncooked eggs to flow underneath. Once the eggs are set, fold the omelet in half and cook for another minute or until fully cooked through. Slide the omelet onto a plate and serve hot, garnished with fresh herbs or a sprinkle of cheese if desired. Enjoy your veggie omelet alongside whole grain toast, fresh fruit, or a side salad for a complete and satisfying breakfast that will fuel your day ahead.

Whole Wheat Pancakes

Whole wheat pancakes offer a nutritious twist on the classic breakfast favorite, providing a hearty and satisfying meal that's packed with fiber, vitamins, and minerals. Made with whole grain flour instead of refined white flour, these pancakes are higher in fiber and nutrients, making them a nutritious option for starting your day.

Here's a comprehensive look at the benefits of whole wheat pancakes and how to make them a delicious and wholesome addition to your breakfast routine:

1. Nutrient-Rich Ingredients: Whole wheat pancakes are made with whole grain flour, which retains the nutrient-rich bran and germ of the wheat kernel. This means that whole wheat pancakes are higher in fiber, vitamins, and minerals compared to traditional pancakes made with refined white flour. Whole wheat flour is an excellent source of dietary fiber, which supports digestive health, regulates blood sugar levels, and promotes feelings of fullness and satiety. Additionally, whole wheat flour contains essential nutrients such as B vitamins, iron, magnesium, and zinc, which are important for overall health and well-being.

2. Heart Health Benefits: Whole wheat pancakes can be part of a heart-healthy diet due to their high fiber content and nutrient-rich ingredients. Dietary fiber has been shown to help lower cholesterol levels, reduce blood pressure, and improve heart health. By choosing whole wheat pancakes instead of pancakes made with refined flour, you can support heart health and reduce the risk of cardiovascular disease. For added heart health benefits, consider topping your whole wheat pancakes with fresh fruit, nuts, or a drizzle of pure maple syrup instead of traditional butter and syrup.

3. Weight Management: Whole wheat pancakes are a filling and satisfying breakfast option that can help support weight management goals. The high fiber content of whole wheat flour helps promote feelings of fullness and satiety, which can prevent overeating and reduce overall calorie intake. Additionally, whole wheat pancakes have a lower glycemic index compared to pancakes made with refined flour, meaning they cause a slower and more gradual increase in blood sugar levels. This can help stabilize blood sugar levels and prevent energy crashes and cravings later in the day, making whole wheat pancakes an excellent choice for those looking to manage their weight.

4. Versatility and Flavor: Whole wheat pancakes are incredibly versatile and can be customized with a variety of toppings and flavorings to suit individual preferences. Add-ins such as fresh or dried fruit, nuts, seeds, spices, and extracts can enhance the flavor and nutritional profile of whole wheat pancakes. Experiment with different combinations to create delicious and satisfying pancake stacks that you'll look forward to enjoying each morning. Whether you prefer classic toppings like berries and maple syrup or more creative combinations like banana-walnut or pumpkin-spice, the possibilities are endless with whole wheat pancakes.

To make whole wheat pancakes, start by whisking together whole wheat flour, baking powder, salt, and any desired spices in a large bowl. In a separate bowl, beat eggs with milk, vanilla extract, and a touch of honey or maple syrup. Combine the wet ingredients with the dry ingredients, stirring until just blended, taking care not to overmix. Then, heat a non-stick skillet or griddle over medium heat and lightly coat it with cooking spray or butter. Pour the pancake batter onto the hot skillet, using a ladle or measuring cup to portion out the batter into evenly sized pancakes. Cook until bubbles form on the surface of the pancakes and the edges begin to look set, then flip and cook for another minute or until golden brown and cooked through. Serve your whole wheat pancakes hot with your favorite toppings and enjoy a nutritious and delicious breakfast that will keep you fueled and satisfied all morning long.

Greek Yogurt Parfait

The Greek yogurt parfait is a popular breakfast option that combines creamy Greek yogurt with layers of fresh fruit, granola, nuts, and seeds for a delicious and nutritious morning treat. Packed with protein, fiber, vitamins, and minerals, the Greek yogurt parfait offers a balanced and satisfying start to the day. Here's a comprehensive look at the benefits of Greek yogurt parfaits and how to make them a delicious and wholesome addition to your breakfast routine:

1. Protein-Rich Base: Greek yogurt serves as the creamy and protein-rich base of the parfait, providing a substantial source of high-quality protein to help keep you full and satisfied until your next meal. Greek yogurt is strained to remove excess whey, resulting in a thicker and creamier texture compared to regular yogurt. This also concentrates the protein content, making Greek yogurt an excellent choice for supporting muscle repair and growth, promoting satiety, and stabilizing blood sugar levels.

2. Calcium and Probiotics: Greek yogurt is also rich in calcium, which is essential for maintaining strong bones and teeth, as well as supporting muscle and nerve function. Additionally, Greek yogurt contains beneficial probiotics, or live bacteria cultures, which promote gut health and digestion. Probiotics help maintain a healthy balance of bacteria in the gut microbiome, which is important for immune function, nutrient absorption, and overall well-being.

3. Fiber-Rich Toppings: The toppings added to the Greek yogurt parfait provide additional flavor, texture, and nutritional benefits. Fresh fruits such as berries, bananas, kiwi, and mango add natural sweetness, vitamins, minerals, and antioxidants to the parfait. Granola, nuts, and seeds add crunch, fiber, healthy fats, and additional protein to the parfait, making it a satisfying and balanced breakfast option.

4. Customizable and Versatile: One of the best things about Greek yogurt parfaits is their versatility and customization options. You can customize your parfait with a variety of fruits, nuts, seeds, and other toppings to suit your taste preferences and dietary needs. Experiment with different flavor combinations and textures to create unique and delicious parfaits that you'll look forward to enjoying each morning.

5. Quick and Easy to Prepare: Greek yogurt parfaits are quick and easy to prepare, making them perfect for busy mornings or on-the-go breakfasts. Simply layer Greek yogurt with your choice of toppings in a glass or bowl, alternating between yogurt, fruits, granola, nuts, and seeds until you reach the top. You can make individual parfaits ahead of time and store them in the refrigerator for a quick and convenient breakfast option throughout the week.

To make a Greek yogurt parfait, start by layering Greek yogurt with fresh fruit, granola, nuts, and seeds in a glass or bowl. Begin with a layer of Greek yogurt at the bottom, followed by a layer of chopped or sliced fruit, then a layer of granola, nuts, or seeds. Repeat the layers until you reach the top of the glass or bowl, then garnish with additional fruit, nuts, or seeds if desired. Serve the Greek yogurt parfait immediately or refrigerate until ready to enjoy. With its creamy texture, protein-rich base, and customizable toppings, the Greek yogurt parfait is a delicious and nutritious breakfast option that's sure to become a favorite in your morning routine.

CHAPTER 5: Lunch Recipe

Grilled Chicken Salad

A grilled chicken salad is a delicious and nutritious meal that combines tender grilled chicken with crisp, fresh vegetables and a flavorful dressing. Packed with protein, fiber, vitamins, and minerals, this salad is not only satisfying but also incredibly versatile, allowing for endless variations to suit individual tastes and dietary preferences. Here's a comprehensive look at the components of a grilled chicken salad and how to create a delicious and wholesome meal:

1. Grilled Chicken: The star of the grilled chicken salad is, of course, the grilled chicken itself. Choose boneless, skinless chicken breasts or thighs and marinate them in your favorite herbs, spices, and marinades for added flavor. Grill the chicken until it's cooked through and has a delicious charred exterior, then slice or chop it into bite-sized pieces to top your salad.

2. Fresh Vegetables: The key to a delicious grilled chicken salad is using fresh, crisp vegetables that add texture, color, and flavor to the dish. Start with a base of leafy greens such as romaine lettuce, spinach, or mixed greens, then add a variety of chopped vegetables such as tomatoes, cucumbers, bell peppers, carrots, and red onions. Feel free to customize your salad with any vegetables you enjoy or have on hand.

3. Additional Toppings: In addition to grilled chicken and fresh vegetables, you can add a variety of toppings to your salad to enhance its flavor and nutrition. Consider adding ingredients such as sliced avocado, crumbled feta or goat cheese, toasted nuts or seeds, dried fruit, or cooked grains like quinoa or farro. These toppings add richness, texture, and additional nutrients to your salad, making it even more satisfying and delicious.

4. Dressing: The dressing is the finishing touch that ties all the flavors of the grilled chicken salad together. Choose a dressing that complements the flavors of the salad, such as a classic vinaigrette, creamy ranch, tangy balsamic, or zesty citrus dressing. You can use store-bought dressing or make your own at home using simple ingredients like olive oil, vinegar, lemon juice, mustard, honey, and herbs.

5. Variations: One of the best things about grilled chicken salad is its versatility and ability to be customized to suit individual preferences. You can switch up the ingredients and flavors to create endless variations of grilled chicken salad, such as a Greek-inspired salad with olives, feta cheese, and tzatziki dressing, or a Southwest-style salad with black beans, corn, avocado, and chipotle ranch dressing.

A grilled chicken salad is a delicious and nutritious meal option that's perfect for lunch or dinner. With tender grilled chicken, crisp fresh vegetables, and a flavorful dressing, it's a satisfying and wholesome dish that's easy to prepare and endlessly customizable. Whether you're looking for a light and refreshing salad or a hearty and filling meal, a grilled chicken salad is sure to please your taste buds and leave you feeling satisfied and nourished.

Quinoa and Vegetable Stir-Fry

Quinoa and Vegetable Stir-Fry: A Nutrient-Packed Meal Option

A quinoa and vegetable stir-fry is a flavorful and nutritious dish that combines protein-rich quinoa with a colorful assortment of fresh vegetables, aromatic herbs, and savory sauces. This vibrant stir-fry offers a balanced combination of complex carbohydrates, plant-based protein, vitamins, minerals, and fiber, making it a wholesome and satisfying meal option. Here's a comprehensive look at the components of a quinoa and vegetable stir-fry and how to create a delicious and nourishing dish:

1. **Quinoa:** Quinoa serves as the nutritious base of the stir-fry, providing a complete source of plant-based protein and essential amino acids. Rinse the quinoa thoroughly before cooking to remove any bitterness, then cook it according to package instructions until fluffy and tender.

Quinoa adds a satisfying chewiness and nutty flavor to the stir-fry, as well as a boost of protein, fiber, iron, and magnesium.

2. Assorted Vegetables: The vegetable component of the stir-fry adds color, texture, and nutrients to the dish. Choose a variety of vegetables such as bell peppers, broccoli, carrots, snap peas, mushrooms, zucchini, and onions. Cut the vegetables into bite-sized pieces for even cooking and vibrant presentation. Vegetables are rich in vitamins, minerals, antioxidants, and dietary fiber, which support overall health and well-being.

3. Aromatic Herbs and Spices: Aromatic herbs and spices add depth of flavor and complexity to the stir-fry. Common ingredients include garlic, ginger, scallions, cilantro, and red chili flakes. Sauté the aromatics in a bit of oil until fragrant before adding the vegetables to the stir-fry. These herbs and spices not only enhance the taste of the dish but also provide additional health benefits such as anti-inflammatory and immune-boosting properties.

4. Sauce: The sauce is the final component that brings all the flavors of the stir-fry together. Choose a sauce that complements the ingredients and flavors of the dish, such as soy sauce, teriyaki sauce, hoisin sauce, or peanut sauce. You can also make your own stir-fry sauce using a combination of soy sauce, rice vinegar, sesame oil, honey or maple syrup, and cornstarch for thickening. Adjust the amount of sauce to your taste preferences, adding more or less as desired.

5. Variations: One of the best things about quinoa and vegetable stir-fry is its versatility and ability to be customized to suit individual preferences. You can switch up the ingredients and flavors to create endless variations of stir-fry, such as a Thai-inspired stir-fry with coconut milk, curry paste, and basil, or a Mediterranean-style stir-fry with olives, sun-dried tomatoes, and feta cheese. Experiment with different combinations of vegetables, sauces, and seasonings to create delicious and unique stir-fry dishes.

A quinoa and vegetable stir-fry is a nutritious and flavorful meal option that's perfect for lunch or dinner. With protein-rich quinoa, an assortment of colorful vegetables, aromatic herbs and spices, and a savory sauce, it's a satisfying and wholesome dish that's easy to prepare and endlessly customizable. Whether you're looking for a quick and healthy weeknight dinner or a creative way to use up leftover vegetables, a quinoa and vegetable stir-fry is sure to please your taste buds and nourish your body.

Black Bean Soup

Black bean soup is a hearty and flavorful dish that offers a satisfying combination of protein, fiber, and nutrients. Made with black beans, aromatic vegetables, savory spices, and a variety of toppings, black bean soup is a comforting and nourishing meal option that's perfect for lunch or dinner. Here's a comprehensive look at the components of black bean soup and how to create a delicious and wholesome dish:

1. Black Beans: The star ingredient of black bean soup is, of course, the black beans themselves. Black beans are a rich source of plant-based protein, fiber, and essential nutrients such as folate, iron, potassium, and magnesium. Rinse and drain canned black beans or soak dried black beans overnight before cooking. Cook the beans until they're tender and creamy, then blend a portion of the beans to create a thick and creamy base for the soup.

2. **Aromatic Vegetables:** Aromatic vegetables such as onions, garlic, carrots, and celery add depth of flavor and aroma to the soup. Sauté the vegetables in a bit of oil until softened and fragrant before adding the beans and broth. This step helps to develop the flavors of the soup and create a rich and savory base.

3. **Savory Spices:** Savory spices and herbs such as cumin, chili powder, paprika, and oregano add warmth, complexity, and depth of flavor to the soup. Adjust the amount of spices to your taste preferences, adding more or less as desired. You can also add a bay leaf or two to the soup while it simmers for added depth of flavor.

4. **Broth:** The broth serves as the liquid component of the soup, adding moisture and

richness to the dish. Use vegetable broth or chicken broth for a flavorful base, or water for a lighter option. You can also use a combination of broth and water for a balance of flavor and texture.

5. Toppings: Toppings add texture, color, and additional flavor to the soup. Common toppings for black bean soup include diced avocado, chopped cilantro, sliced green onions, sour cream or Greek yogurt, shredded cheese, and crushed tortilla chips or strips. Garnish the soup with your favorite toppings just before serving for a fresh and vibrant finishing touch.

Black bean soup is a delicious and nutritious meal option that's easy to prepare and full of flavor. With protein-rich black beans, aromatic vegetables, savory spices, and a variety of toppings, it's a satisfying and wholesome dish that's perfect for cozying up on a chilly day or enjoying as a light and healthy meal any time of year. Whether you prefer a classic version of black bean soup or want to experiment with different ingredients and flavors, there are endless possibilities for creating delicious and nourishing variations of this comforting soup.

Turkey Wrap with Lettuce

The turkey wrap with lettuce is a delicious and nutritious meal option that combines lean turkey breast with crisp lettuce leaves and a variety of flavorful fillings. This versatile dish is perfect for lunch or a light dinner, offering a satisfying balance of protein, fiber, vitamins, and minerals. Here's a comprehensive look at the components of a turkey wrap with lettuce and how to create a delicious and wholesome meal:

1. Lean Turkey Breast: The key ingredient of the turkey wrap is lean turkey breast, which provides a lean source of protein that's low in fat and calories. Choose sliced deli turkey breast or cooked turkey breast slices for convenience, or roast a turkey breast at home for added flavor. Turkey breast is rich in protein, which is essential for muscle repair, growth, and maintenance, as well as supporting overall health and well-being.

2. Crisp Lettuce Leaves: Crisp lettuce leaves serve as the base of the wrap, providing a refreshing and crunchy texture that contrasts with the tender turkey breast. Choose sturdy lettuce varieties such as romaine, iceberg, or leaf lettuce, which can hold up well to the fillings without becoming soggy. Alternatively, you can use large leaves of butter lettuce or Boston lettuce for a softer and more delicate wrap.

3. Flavorful Fillings: The fillings of the turkey wrap add flavor, texture, and nutrition to the dish. Common fillings include sliced tomatoes, cucumbers, bell peppers, avocado, red onion, and shredded carrots. You can also add spreads such as hummus, mustard, or pesto for added flavor and moisture. Experiment with different combinations of fillings to create a wrap that suits your taste preferences and dietary needs.

4. Assembly: To assemble the turkey wrap, start by laying a lettuce leaf flat on a clean surface. Place slices of turkey breast on top of the lettuce leaf, then add your desired fillings on top of the turkey. Roll up the lettuce leaf tightly around the fillings to form a wrap, tucking in the sides as you go to enclose the fillings securely. Repeat with additional lettuce leaves and fillings to make as many wraps as desired.

5. Variations: The beauty of the turkey wrap with lettuce is its versatility and ability to be customized to suit individual preferences. You can switch up the ingredients and flavors to create endless variations of wraps, such as a Greek-inspired wrap with feta cheese, olives, and tzatziki sauce, or a Tex-Mex wrap with black beans, salsa, and shredded cheese. Get creative and have fun experimenting with different combinations of fillings to create delicious and satisfying turkey wraps that you'll love to enjoy for lunch or dinner.

The turkey wrap with lettuce is a nutritious and delicious meal option that's perfect for a quick and easy lunch or dinner. With lean turkey breast, crisp lettuce leaves, and a variety of flavorful fillings, it's a satisfying and wholesome dish that's easy to prepare and endlessly customizable. Whether you prefer a classic turkey and vegetable wrap or want to experiment with different ingredients and flavors, the turkey wrap with lettuce offers endless possibilities for creating delicious and nourishing meals that you'll enjoy time and time again.

CHAPTER 6: Dinner Recipes

Baked Salmon with Lemon

Baked salmon with lemon is a flavorful and nutritious dish that combines tender salmon fillets with zesty lemon flavor for a delicious and satisfying meal. Salmon is a rich source of omega-3 fatty acids, protein, vitamins, and minerals, while lemon adds brightness and acidity to enhance the natural flavors of the fish. Here's a comprehensive look at the components of baked salmon with lemon and how to create a mouthwatering dish:

1. Salmon: Choose high-quality salmon fillets for the best results. Wild-caught salmon is preferred for its superior flavor and nutritional profile, although farm-raised salmon can also be delicious when sourced responsibly. Salmon is rich in omega-3 fatty acids, which are beneficial for heart health, brain function, and reducing inflammation. It is also an excellent source of protein, vitamin D, and B vitamins.

2. Lemon: Fresh lemon juice and zest are essential for adding brightness and acidity to the baked salmon. Lemon not only enhances the flavor of the fish but also helps to tenderize the flesh and keep it moist during cooking. The acidic nature of lemon juice also helps to balance the richness of the salmon and cut through any fishy taste. Be sure to use freshly squeezed lemon juice and finely grated lemon zest for the best results.

3. Seasonings: In addition to lemon, season the salmon filets with a combination of herbs, spices, and aromatics to add depth of flavor. Common seasonings for baked salmon include minced garlic, fresh dill, parsley, thyme, and black pepper. You can also add a sprinkle of sea salt or a drizzle of olive oil for extra flavor and moisture.

4. Baking Method: Preheat the oven to the desired temperature, usually around 375°F to 400°F. Place the salmon fillets on a baking sheet lined with parchment paper or aluminum foil for easy cleanup. Drizzle the fillets with lemon juice and olive oil, then sprinkle with the desired seasonings. Bake the salmon in the preheated oven for about 12-15 minutes, or until the fish is opaque and flakes easily with a fork.

5. Garnishes: Garnish the baked salmon with additional lemon slices or wedges for serving. Fresh herbs such as dill or parsley can also be added for a pop of color and freshness. Serve the baked salmon hot alongside your favorite side dishes, such as roasted vegetables, steamed rice, or a crisp salad, for a complete and satisfying meal.

Baked salmon with lemon is a simple yet elegant dish that's perfect for any occasion. With its tender, flavorful fish and bright, zesty lemon flavor, it's a healthy and delicious meal option that's sure to impress. Whether you're cooking for a special dinner or a quick weeknight meal, baked salmon with lemon is a versatile and satisfying choice that's sure to become a favorite in your recipe repertoire.

Roasted Chicken Breast with Vegetables

Roasted chicken breast with vegetables is a classic and comforting dish that combines tender chicken breast with an assortment of colorful vegetables for a flavorful and nutritious meal. This versatile dish is easy to prepare and can be customized with a variety of herbs, spices, and seasonings to suit individual tastes. Here's a comprehensive look at the components of roasted chicken breast with vegetables and how to create a delicious and wholesome meal:

1. Chicken Breast: Start with boneless, skinless chicken breasts for a lean and healthy protein source. Chicken breast is low in fat and calories but high in protein, making it an excellent choice for those looking to maintain a balanced diet. Season the chicken breasts with your favorite herbs and spices, such as garlic powder, onion powder, paprika, thyme, rosemary, or Italian seasoning, for added flavor.

2. Assorted Vegetables: Choose a variety of fresh vegetables to accompany the chicken breast in the roasting pan. Popular options include bell peppers, onions, carrots, zucchini, squash, broccoli, cauliflower, cherry tomatoes, and Brussels sprouts. Cut the vegetables into bite-sized pieces or wedges and toss them with olive oil, salt, pepper, and any desired seasonings before adding them to the roasting pan.

3. Roasting Method: Preheat the oven to the desired temperature, typically around 400°F to 425°F. Place the seasoned chicken breasts and prepared vegetables on a large baking sheet or roasting pan lined with parchment paper or aluminum foil for easy cleanup. Arrange the chicken breasts in the center of the pan and surround them with the vegetables. Drizzle everything with olive oil and sprinkle with additional seasonings, if desired.

4. Cooking Time: Roast the chicken breasts and vegetables in the preheated oven for about 20-25 minutes, or until the chicken is cooked through and the vegetables are tender and caramelized. The exact cooking time may vary depending on the thickness of the chicken breasts and the types of vegetables used, so it's important to monitor the dish closely to prevent overcooking.

5. Serve and Enjoy: Once the chicken breasts and vegetables are cooked to perfection, remove them from the oven and let them rest for a few minutes before serving. Slice the chicken breasts crosswise and divide them among plates, along with generous portions of the roasted vegetables. Garnish with fresh herbs, such as parsley or basil, and serve hot as a delicious and satisfying meal.

Roasted chicken breast with vegetables is a wholesome and flavorful dish that's perfect for any occasion. With its tender, juicy chicken and vibrant, caramelized vegetables, it's a satisfying and nutritious meal option that's easy to prepare and sure to please the whole family. Whether you're cooking for a weeknight dinner or a special gathering, roasted chicken breast with vegetables is a versatile and delicious choice that's sure to become a favorite in your recipe repertoire.

Cauliflower Fried Rice

Cauliflower fried rice is a delicious and nutritious alternative to traditional fried rice that substitutes cauliflower rice for rice grains. This low-carb, gluten-free dish is packed with flavor and loaded with vegetables, making it a satisfying and healthy meal option. Here's a comprehensive look at the components of cauliflower fried rice and how to create a delicious and wholesome dish:

1. Cauliflower Rice: The base of cauliflower fried rice is cauliflower rice, which is simply cauliflower florets that have been grated or processed into small, rice-like pieces. Cauliflower rice is a low-carb alternative to traditional rice, making it perfect for those following a keto or paleo diet or looking to reduce their carbohydrate intake. You can make cauliflower rice at home by grating a head of cauliflower using a box grater or food processor, or purchase pre-made cauliflower rice from the grocery store for added convenience.

2. Assorted Vegetables: Cauliflower fried rice is loaded with an assortment of colorful vegetables, adding flavor, texture, and nutrition to the dish. Common vegetables used in cauliflower fried rice include onions, garlic, carrots, bell peppers, peas, corn, broccoli, and green onions. Chop the vegetables into small, uniform pieces for even cooking and distribution throughout the dish.

3. Protein: Add protein to your cauliflower fried rice by incorporating cooked chicken, shrimp, tofu, or eggs. You can cook the protein separately and add it to the fried rice towards the end of cooking, or cook it directly in the same skillet or wok along with the vegetables. Protein adds satiety and helps to make the dish more filling and satisfying.

4. Seasonings and Sauces: Season cauliflower fried rice with a combination of spices, herbs, and sauces to enhance the flavor of the dish. Common seasonings and sauces used in cauliflower fried rice include soy sauce, sesame oil, ginger, garlic, chili paste, and rice vinegar. Adjust the amount of seasoning and sauce to your taste preferences, adding more or less as desired.

5. Cooking Method: To make cauliflower fried rice, start by sautéing the vegetables in a bit of oil until they're softened and fragrant. Add the cauliflower rice to the skillet or wok and cook until it's tender but not mushy, stirring frequently to ensure even cooking. Push the cauliflower rice and vegetables to the side of the skillet or wok and scramble the eggs in the empty space until they're cooked through. Finally, add the protein and any additional seasonings or sauces to the skillet or wok and toss everything together until well combined and heated through.

Cauliflower fried rice is a delicious and nutritious dish that's easy to make and perfect for a quick weeknight dinner or meal prep. With its flavorful cauliflower rice, colorful vegetables, protein-rich additions, and savory seasonings, it's a satisfying and wholesome meal option that's sure to become a favorite in your recipe repertoire. Whether you're looking for a low-carb alternative to traditional fried rice or simply want to incorporate more vegetables into your diet, cauliflower fried rice is a versatile and delicious choice that's sure to please your taste buds and nourish your body.

Spaghetti Squash with Marinara Sauce

Spaghetti squash with marinara sauce is a delicious and nutritious alternative to traditional pasta dishes, offering a lighter and lower-carb option that's packed with flavor and nutrients. Spaghetti squash, when cooked, has a unique texture that resembles spaghetti noodles, making it a versatile and satisfying base for a variety of sauces and toppings. Here's a comprehensive look at the components of spaghetti squash with marinara sauce and how to create a delicious and wholesome dish:

1. Spaghetti Squash: Spaghetti squash is a winter squash variety known for its stringy flesh, which separates into spaghetti-like strands when cooked. To prepare spaghetti squash, start by cutting it in half lengthwise and removing the seeds and pulp. Roast the squash halves in the oven until tender, then use a fork to scrape out the strands of cooked squash, which will resemble spaghetti noodles. Spaghetti squash is low in calories and carbohydrates, high in fiber, and rich in vitamins and minerals, making it a nutritious alternative to traditional pasta.

2. Marinara Sauce: Marinara sauce is a classic Italian tomato-based sauce that's rich in flavor and versatile in its use. To make marinara sauce, start by sautéing aromatics such as onions, garlic, and herbs in olive oil until softened and fragrant. Add canned crushed tomatoes, tomato paste, and additional seasonings such as salt, pepper, oregano, basil, and red pepper flakes. Simmer the sauce until it thickens and the flavors meld together, then adjust the seasonings to taste. Marinara sauce is a delicious and healthy option for topping spaghetti squash, providing a burst of flavor and nutrients without the excess calories or fat found in cream-based sauces.

3. Toppings and Additions: Spaghetti squash with marinara sauce can be customized with a variety of toppings and additions to suit individual tastes. Consider adding cooked protein such as grilled chicken, shrimp, or Italian sausage for added flavor and satiety. You can also top the dish with grated Parmesan cheese, chopped fresh herbs such as basil or parsley, or a sprinkle of red pepper flakes for heat. Serve the spaghetti squash with marinara sauce hot and garnish with your favorite toppings for a satisfying and nutritious meal.

4. Variations: Spaghetti squash with marinara sauce can be customized in endless ways to create unique and delicious variations of the dish. Try adding sautéed vegetables such as mushrooms, bell peppers, or spinach to the marinara sauce for added flavor and nutrition. You can also experiment with different types of sauces, such as pesto, Alfredo, or vodka sauce, for a change of pace. Get creative and have fun experimenting with different toppings, additions, and flavor combinations to create a spaghetti squash dish that's perfect for your palate.

Spaghetti squash with marinara sauce is a delicious and nutritious dish that's perfect for anyone looking to enjoy a lighter and healthier alternative to traditional pasta dishes. With its tender spaghetti squash noodles, flavorful marinara sauce, and endless customization options, it's a satisfying and wholesome meal option that's sure to please the whole family.

Whether you're looking for a quick and easy weeknight dinner or a nutritious and comforting meal to enjoy any time, spaghetti squash with marinara sauce is a versatile and delicious choice that's sure to become a favorite in your recipe repertoire.

CHAPTER 7: Snack Ideas

Apple Slices with Peanut Butter

Apple slices with peanut butter is a delicious and nutritious snack that combines the natural sweetness of apples with the rich creaminess of peanut butter for a satisfying and wholesome treat. This simple yet flavorful snack is not only delicious but also provides a good balance of carbohydrates, protein, healthy fats, fiber, vitamins, and minerals. Here's a comprehensive look at the components of apple slices with peanut butter and how to create a delicious and nutritious snack:

1. Apples: Apples are a versatile and nutritious fruit that serves as the perfect base for this snack. Choose your favorite variety of apple, such as Granny Smith, Gala, Honeycrisp, or Fuji, depending on your taste preferences. Apples are rich in fiber, vitamin C, antioxidants, and various other nutrients that support overall health and well-being. Wash the apples thoroughly and slice them into wedges or rounds for easy dipping.

2. Peanut Butter: Peanut butter is a creamy and delicious spread made from ground peanuts, often mixed with a touch of salt and sometimes sweeteners. Opt for natural peanut butter without added sugars or hydrogenated oils for the healthiest option. Peanut butter is a good source of protein, healthy fats, and essential nutrients such as vitamin E, magnesium, and potassium. Spread a dollop of peanut butter onto each apple slice, or use it as a dip for dunking the apple slices.

3. Nutritional Benefits: Apple slices with peanut butter offer a combination of carbohydrates from the apples, protein from the peanut butter, and healthy fats from the peanuts. This combination provides sustained energy, helps to stabilize blood sugar levels, and keeps you feeling full and satisfied between meals. The fiber in both the apples and peanut butter aids in digestion and promotes gut health, while the vitamins and minerals contribute to overall wellness.

4. Variations: While classic peanut butter is a delicious choice for apple slices, you can also experiment with other nut or seed butters such as almond butter, cashew butter, or sunflower seed butter for different flavor profiles and nutritional benefits. For added texture and flavor, you can sprinkle the peanut butter-topped apple slices with toppings such as chopped nuts, granola, cinnamon, or dark chocolate chips.

5. Enjoyment: Apple slices with peanut butter make for a convenient and portable snack that's perfect for enjoying on the go or at home. Whether you're craving a mid-afternoon pick-me-up, a pre-workout snack, or a simple dessert, apple slices with peanut butter are a satisfying and nutritious choice that's sure to please your taste buds and keep you feeling energized and nourished throughout the day.

Apple slices with peanut butter are a delicious and nutritious snack that's easy to prepare and perfect for satisfying hunger cravings any time of day. With their natural sweetness, crisp texture, and creamy richness, apple slices paired with peanut butter offer a delightful combination of flavors and textures that's both satisfying and nourishing. Whether you're enjoying them as a quick snack, a pre- or post-workout fuel, or a simple dessert, apple slices with peanut butter are sure to become a favorite go-to snack in your healthy eating repertoire.

Celery Sticks with Hummus

Celery sticks with hummus is a nutritious and satisfying snack that combines crunchy celery with creamy hummus for a delicious and wholesome treat. This simple yet flavorful snack is not only delicious but also provides a good balance of carbohydrates, protein, healthy fats, fiber, vitamins, and minerals. Here's a comprehensive look at the components of celery sticks with hummus and how to create a delicious and nutritious snack:

1. Celery Sticks: Celery is a crisp and refreshing vegetable that serves as the perfect vessel for scooping up creamy hummus. It is low in calories and carbohydrates but rich in fiber, vitamin K, and antioxidants. Wash the celery thoroughly and cut it into manageable sticks for easy dipping. Celery sticks offer a satisfying crunch and a mild, slightly sweet flavor that compliments the savory taste of hummus.

2. Hummus: Hummus is a creamy spread made from cooked and mashed chickpeas (garbanzo beans), blended with tahini (sesame seed paste), olive oil, lemon juice, garlic, and salt. It is rich in protein, healthy fats, fiber, and essential nutrients such as folate, iron, and magnesium. Choose traditional hummus or experiment with different flavors such as roasted red pepper, garlic and herb, or spicy jalapeno for added variety and flavor. Hummus provides a creamy and flavorful dip that pairs perfectly with the crispness of celery sticks.

3. Nutritional Benefits: Celery sticks with hummus offer a combination of carbohydrates from the celery, protein and healthy fats from the hummus, and fiber from both components. This combination provides sustained energy, helps to stabilize blood sugar levels, and keeps you feeling full and satisfied between meals. The fiber in both the celery and hummus aids in digestion and promotes gut health, while the vitamins and minerals contribute to overall wellness.

4. Variations: While classic hummus is a delicious choice for celery sticks, you can also experiment with other bean-based dips such as black bean dip, white bean dip, or edamame dip for different flavor profiles and nutritional benefits. For added texture and flavor, you can sprinkle the hummus-topped celery sticks with toppings such as chopped fresh herbs, toasted sesame seeds, paprika, or a drizzle of extra virgin olive oil.

5. Enjoyment: Celery sticks with hummus make for a convenient and portable snack that's perfect for enjoying on the go or at home. Whether you're craving a mid-afternoon pick-me-up, a pre-workout snack, or a simple appetizer, celery sticks with hummus are a satisfying and nutritious choice that's sure to please your taste buds and keep you feeling energized and nourished throughout the day.

Celery sticks with hummus are a delicious and nutritious snack that's easy to prepare and perfect for satisfying hunger cravings any time of day. With their crisp texture, mild flavor, and creamy richness, celery sticks paired with hummus offer a delightful combination of flavors and textures that's both satisfying and nourishing. Whether you're enjoying them as a quick snack, a pre- or post-workout fuel, or a simple appetizer, celery sticks with hummus are sure to become a favorite go-to snack in your healthy eating repertoire.

Mixed Nuts and Seeds

Mixed nuts and seeds are a nutritious and satisfying snack that combines a variety of nuts and seeds for a delicious and wholesome treat. This simple yet flavorful snack is not only delicious but also provides a good balance of protein, healthy fats, fiber, vitamins, and minerals. Here's a comprehensive look at the components of mixed nuts and seeds and how to create a delicious and nutritious snack:

1. Nuts: Nuts such as almonds, walnuts, cashews, pecans, and pistachios are rich in protein, healthy fats, fiber, vitamins, and minerals. Each type of nut offers a unique nutritional profile, with almonds being high in vitamin E and magnesium, walnuts being rich in omega-3 fatty acids, cashews being a good source of iron and zinc, pecans being high in antioxidants, and pistachios being rich in potassium and vitamin B6. Choose raw or dry-roasted nuts without added salt or sugar for the healthiest option.

2. Seeds: Seeds such as pumpkin seeds, sunflower seeds, flaxseeds, chia seeds, and hemp seeds are also packed with protein, healthy fats, fiber, vitamins, and minerals. Pumpkin seeds are rich in magnesium and zinc, sunflower seeds are high in vitamin E and selenium, flaxseeds are a good source of omega-3 fatty acids and lignans, chia seeds are high in fiber and omega-3 fatty acids, and hemp seeds are rich in protein and essential fatty acids. Seeds add texture and crunch to the mixed nuts and seeds snack and offer a variety of health benefits.

3. Nutritional Benefits: Mixed nuts and seeds offer a combination of protein, healthy fats, fiber, vitamins, and minerals that provide sustained energy, help to stabilize blood sugar levels, and keep you feeling full and satisfied between meals. The protein and healthy fats in mixed nuts and seeds promote satiety and help to curb cravings, while the fiber aids in digestion and promotes gut health. The vitamins and minerals in mixed nuts and seeds support overall health and well-being, including immune function, heart health, and bone health.

4. Variations: You can customize mixed nuts and seeds according to your taste preferences and dietary needs by mixing and matching different types of nuts and seeds. Consider adding dried fruits such as raisins, cranberries, or apricots for added sweetness and flavor, or spices such as cinnamon, cayenne pepper, or curry powder for added warmth and depth of flavor. You can also roast the nuts and seeds with a touch of honey or maple syrup for a deliciously sweet and crunchy snack.

5. Portion Control: While mixed nuts and seeds are a nutritious snack, it's important to practice portion control, as they are calorie-dense foods. A serving size of mixed nuts and seeds is typically about a quarter cup or a small handful, which provides a good balance of nutrients without going overboard on calories. Enjoy mixed nuts and seeds as a snack on their own, or add them to yogurt, oatmeal, salads, or trail mix for added texture and flavor.

Mixed nuts and seeds are a delicious and nutritious snack that's easy to prepare and perfect for satisfying hunger cravings any time of day. With their crunchy texture, rich flavor, and diverse nutritional benefits, mixed nuts and seeds offer a delightful combination of flavors and textures that's both satisfying and nourishing. Whether you're enjoying them as a quick snack on the go, a pre- or post-workout fuel, or a nutritious addition to your meals, mixed nuts and seeds are sure to become a favorite go-to snack in your healthy eating repertoire.

Cottage Cheese and Berries

Cottage cheese and berries is a nutritious and delicious snack or meal option that combines creamy cottage cheese with fresh or frozen berries for a satisfying and wholesome treat. This simple yet flavorful combination is not only tasty but also provides a good balance of protein, carbohydrates, fiber, vitamins, and minerals.

Here's a comprehensive look at the components of cottage cheese and berries and how to create a delicious and nutritious snack:

1. Cottage Cheese: Cottage cheese is a fresh cheese made from curds of pasteurized cow's milk. It is rich in protein, low in fat, and provides essential nutrients such as calcium, phosphorus, and selenium. Cottage cheese is known for its creamy texture and mild flavor, making it a versatile ingredient in both sweet and savory dishes. Opt for low-fat or non-fat varieties of cottage cheese for a healthier option. Cottage cheese provides a creamy and protein-rich base for the snack, helping to keep you feeling full and satisfied.

2. Berries: Berries such as strawberries, blueberries, raspberries, and blackberries are rich in antioxidants, vitamins, and fiber. They are low in calories and carbohydrates but high in flavor and nutrition, making them the perfect complement to creamy cottage cheese. Berries are naturally sweet and juicy, adding a burst of color, freshness, and sweetness to the snack. Choose fresh berries when they're in season or opt for frozen berries for convenience and year-round availability.

3. Nutritional Benefits: Cottage cheese and berries offer a combination of protein, carbohydrates, fiber, vitamins, and minerals that provide sustained energy, help to stabilize blood sugar levels, and keep you feeling full and satisfied between meals. The protein in cottage cheese promotes satiety and helps to curb cravings, while the fiber in berries aids in digestion and promotes gut health. Berries are also rich in antioxidants, which help to protect against oxidative stress and inflammation in the body.

4. Variations: You can customize cottage cheese and berries according to your taste preferences and dietary needs by experimenting with different types of berries and cottage cheese varieties. Consider adding a drizzle of honey or maple syrup for added sweetness, or sprinkle the snack with chopped nuts or seeds for added texture and flavor. You can also blend cottage cheese and berries together to create a creamy and delicious smoothie or parfait.

5. Portion Control: While cottage cheese and berries are a nutritious snack, it's important to practice portion control to avoid overeating. A serving size of cottage cheese is typically about half a cup, while a serving size of berries is about one cup. Aim to fill your bowl or plate with a balance of cottage cheese and berries, keeping in mind your individual calorie and nutrient needs. Enjoy cottage cheese and berries as a satisfying and nutritious snack, breakfast, or dessert that's perfect for any time of day.

Cottage cheese and berries is a delicious and nutritious snack or meal option that's easy to prepare and perfect for satisfying hunger cravings any time of day. With its creamy texture, sweet and juicy berries, and diverse nutritional benefits, cottage cheese and berries offer a delightful combination of flavors and textures that's both satisfying and nourishing. Whether you're enjoying it as a quick snack on the go, a light breakfast, or a refreshing dessert, cottage cheese and berries are sure to become a favorite go-to option in your healthy eating repertoire.

CHAPTER 8. Dessert Recipes

Sugar-Free Chocolate Mousse

Sugar-free chocolate mousse is a decadent and indulgent dessert that provides all the rich and creamy goodness of traditional chocolate mousse without the added sugar. This delicious treat is perfect for those looking to satisfy their sweet tooth while still adhering to a low-sugar or sugar-free diet. Here's a comprehensive look at the components of sugar-free chocolate mousse and how to create a delicious and guilt-free dessert:

1. Chocolate: Start with high-quality dark chocolate or sugar-free chocolate chips as the base for your mousse. Dark chocolate contains less sugar than milk chocolate and is rich in antioxidants, which may offer various health benefits, including improved heart health and brain function. Opt for chocolate with a cocoa content of at least 70% for the best flavor and nutritional value. You can also use sugar-free chocolate chips sweetened with alternative sweeteners such as stevia or erythritol for a completely sugar-free option.

2. Cream: Heavy cream or whipping cream is essential for creating the creamy texture of chocolate mousse. Choose a high-fat cream for the best results, as it will whip up into a light and fluffy consistency. Be sure to chill the cream before whipping it to ensure that it holds its shape and forms stiff peaks when whipped. You can also use coconut cream or almond milk for a dairy-free alternative.

3. Sweetener: Instead of traditional granulated sugar, use a sugar-free sweetener such as stevia, erythritol, monk fruit, or xylitol to sweeten the chocolate mousse. These sweeteners provide the sweetness you crave without the added calories or impact on blood sugar levels. Adjust the amount of sweetener to taste, adding more or less as desired to achieve your preferred level of sweetness.

4. Flavorings: Enhance the flavor of the chocolate mousse with a splash of vanilla extract or a pinch of sea salt. Vanilla extract adds a subtle sweetness and depth of flavor, while sea salt helps to balance the sweetness and intensify the chocolate flavor. You can also experiment with other flavorings such as almond extract, peppermint extract, or espresso powder for added complexity and depth.

5. Texture: To achieve the perfect texture for sugar-free chocolate mousse, it's important to properly melt the chocolate and whip the cream to stiff peaks before folding them together. Melt the chocolate gently using a double boiler or in the microwave, being careful not to overheat it. Once melted, let the chocolate cool slightly before folding it into the whipped cream to avoid deflating the mixture. Gently fold the chocolate into the whipped cream until fully incorporated, being careful not to overmix.

6. Chilling: After assembling the chocolate mousse, transfer it to individual serving dishes or a large bowl and chill it in the refrigerator for at least a few hours, or until set. Chilling allows the mousse to firm up and develop its rich and creamy texture. For best results, chill the mousse overnight to allow the flavors to meld together and intensify.

Sugar-free chocolate mousse is a delicious and guilt-free dessert that's perfect for satisfying your sweet cravings without the added sugar. With its rich chocolate flavor, creamy texture, and indulgent taste, sugar-free chocolate mousse is sure to become a favorite treat for anyone looking to enjoy a healthier alternative to traditional desserts. Whether you're following a low-sugar or sugar-free diet or simply looking for a delicious and satisfying dessert option, sugar-free chocolate mousse is a delightful choice that's sure to please your taste buds and leave you feeling satisfied and guilt-free.

Berry Crumble

Berry crumble is a delightful and comforting dessert that showcases the natural sweetness and vibrant flavors of fresh or frozen berries, topped with a crunchy and buttery crumble topping. This classic dessert is easy to make and perfect for showcasing seasonal fruits while providing a deliciously satisfying treat. Here's a comprehensive look at the components of berry crumble and how to create a delicious and wholesome dessert:

1. Berries: The star of berry crumble is, of course, the berries. Choose your favorite combination of fresh or frozen berries, such as strawberries, blueberries, raspberries, blackberries, or a mixture of all. Berries are rich in antioxidants, vitamins, and fiber, making them a nutritious and flavorful choice for this dessert. They provide natural sweetness and juiciness to the crumble, bursting with flavor with every bite.

2. Crumble Topping: The crumble topping is made from a mixture of flour, oats, sugar, butter, and spices. Flour and oats provide the base for the crumble, while sugar adds sweetness and helps to caramelize the topping during baking. Butter is used to bind the ingredients together and create a crumbly texture, while spices such as cinnamon, nutmeg, or cardamom add warmth and depth of flavor. You can also add chopped nuts or seeds for extra crunch and texture.

3. Assembly: To assemble the berry crumble, start by tossing the berries with a bit of sugar and cornstarch to thicken the juices. Arrange the berries in a baking dish or individual ramekins, then sprinkle the crumble topping evenly over the top. Gently pat down the topping to ensure even coverage. Bake the crumble in a preheated oven until the berries are bubbling and the topping is golden brown and crisp.

4. Variations: Berry crumble is highly versatile and can be customized according to personal taste preferences and dietary needs. You can experiment with different combinations of berries, or add other fruits such as apples, peaches, or rhubarb for added flavor and variety. For a healthier twist, you can use whole grain flour, coconut sugar, or a sugar alternative such as maple syrup or honey in place of refined sugar. You can also add spices such as ginger, cloves, or allspice for a unique and aromatic flavor profile.

5. Serving: Serve berry crumble warm out of the oven, topped with a scoop of vanilla ice cream or a dollop of whipped cream for an extra indulgent treat. Alternatively, enjoy it plain or with a drizzle of honey or maple syrup for added sweetness. Berry crumble is perfect for any occasion, whether it's a cozy family dinner, a weekend brunch, or a special celebration. It's a comforting and satisfying dessert that's sure to please everyone's taste buds.

Berry crumble is a delicious and comforting dessert that's perfect for showcasing the natural sweetness and flavors of fresh or frozen berries. With its juicy fruit filling and crunchy crumble topping, berry crumble offers a delightful contrast of textures and flavors that's sure to satisfy any sweet tooth. Whether you're enjoying it on its own or with a scoop of ice cream, berry crumble is a timeless dessert that's sure to become a favorite in your recipe repertoire.

Avocado Chocolate Pudding

Avocado chocolate pudding is a creamy and decadent dessert that offers a healthy twist by incorporating nutrient-rich avocado as the main ingredient. This delicious treat provides all the richness and indulgence of traditional chocolate pudding while adding the creamy texture and health benefits of avocado. Here's a comprehensive look at the components of avocado chocolate pudding and how to create a delicious and nutritious dessert:

1. Avocado: Avocado serves as the creamy base for this pudding, providing a velvety texture and subtle flavor that pairs perfectly with chocolate. Avocado is rich in heart-healthy monounsaturated fats, fiber, vitamins, and minerals. It adds creaminess to the pudding while also providing essential nutrients that support overall health and well-being. Choose ripe avocados that are soft to the touch and free from bruises or blemishes for the best results.

2. Chocolate: High-quality cocoa powder or melted dark chocolate is used to add rich chocolate flavor to the pudding. Cocoa powder is rich in antioxidants and flavonoids, which have been linked to various health benefits, including improved heart health and cognitive function. Dark chocolate contains less sugar than milk chocolate and provides a more intense chocolate flavor. Opt for unsweetened cocoa powder or dark chocolate with a cocoa content of at least 70% for the best flavor and nutritional value.

3. Sweetener: To sweeten the avocado chocolate pudding, use a natural sweetener such as maple syrup, honey, agave nectar, or dates. These sweeteners provide sweetness without the added sugars found in traditional pudding recipes, making them a healthier option. Adjust the amount of sweetener to taste, adding more or less as desired to achieve your preferred level of sweetness.

4. Flavorings: Enhance the flavor of the avocado chocolate pudding with a splash of vanilla extract or a pinch of sea salt. Vanilla extract adds a subtle sweetness and depth of flavor, while sea salt helps to balance the sweetness and intensify the chocolate flavor. You can also add other flavorings such as almond extract, peppermint extract, or espresso powder for added complexity and depth.

5. Texture: To achieve the perfect texture for avocado chocolate pudding, blend the avocado, cocoa powder or melted chocolate, sweetener, and flavorings together in a food processor or blender until smooth and creamy. Adjust the consistency by adding a splash of milk or dairy-free milk alternative as needed to achieve your desired thickness. Chill the pudding in the refrigerator for at least a few hours, or until set, before serving.

Avocado chocolate pudding is a delicious and nutritious dessert that's perfect for satisfying your sweet cravings while also providing essential nutrients and health benefits. With its creamy texture, rich chocolate flavor, and wholesome ingredients, avocado chocolate pudding is sure to become a favorite treat for anyone looking to enjoy a healthier alternative to traditional desserts. Whether you're following a plant-based diet, trying to incorporate more nutrient-rich foods into your diet, or simply looking for a delicious and satisfying dessert option, avocado chocolate pudding is a delightful choice that's sure to please your taste buds and leave you feeling satisfied and nourished.

Coconut Macaroons

Coconut macaroons are delightful and indulgent treats that boast a perfect balance of chewy texture, sweet flavor, and tropical aroma. These bite-sized delights are typically made from shredded coconut, egg whites, sugar, and vanilla extract, offering a simple yet irresistible dessert option. Here's a comprehensive look at the components of coconut macaroons and how to create a delicious batch:

1. Shredded Coconut: The star ingredient of coconut macaroons is shredded coconut, which provides the signature flavor and texture. Unsweetened shredded coconut is typically used, although sweetened varieties can also be incorporated for added sweetness. The coconut adds a chewy and moist texture to the macaroons while infusing them with its distinct tropical flavor.

2. Egg Whites: Egg whites serve as the binding agent in coconut macaroons, helping to hold the ingredients together and giving the macaroons their light and airy texture. When whipped to stiff peaks, egg whites create a fluffy and meringue-like consistency that contributes to the macaroons' delicate structure.

3. Sugar: Sugar is added to coconut macaroons to provide sweetness and enhance the flavor profile. Granulated sugar or confectioners' sugar can be used, depending on personal preference. Some recipes also call for sweetened condensed milk, which adds sweetness and richness to the macaroons.

4. Vanilla Extract: Vanilla extract is often included in coconut macaroon recipes to add depth of flavor and aroma. It complements the sweetness of the coconut and sugar, providing a subtle yet enticing undertone to the finished product.

5. Baking Process: To make coconut macaroons, the shredded coconut is combined with whipped egg whites, sugar, and vanilla extract to form a sticky dough. The dough is then scooped into small mounds and placed on a baking sheet lined with parchment paper. The macaroons are baked in a preheated oven until they are golden brown and lightly crisp on the outside while remaining soft and chewy on the inside.

6. Variations: While classic coconut macaroons are simple and delicious on their own, there are endless variations and flavor combinations to explore. Consider dipping the baked macaroons in melted chocolate for added decadence, or incorporating chopped nuts, dried fruit, or citrus zest for extra texture and flavor. You can also experiment with different extracts such as almond, coconut, or lemon to create unique and flavorful variations of this beloved dessert.

Coconut macaroons are a delightful and versatile treat that's perfect for satisfying sweet cravings and indulging in a taste of the tropics. With their chewy texture, sweet coconut flavor, and endless variations, coconut macaroons are sure to become a favorite dessert option for any occasion. Whether enjoyed on their own or as part of a dessert platter, coconut macaroons offer a simple yet irresistible treat that's sure to please everyone's palate.

CHAPTER 9. Tips for Dining Out

Choosing Healthy Options

Choosing healthy options is essential for maintaining overall well-being and supporting a balanced lifestyle. Whether it's selecting nutritious foods, engaging in regular physical activity, or prioritizing self-care practices, making healthy choices plays a crucial role in promoting optimal health. Here's a comprehensive look at various aspects of choosing healthy options and their importance:

1. Nutritious Foods: Opting for nutrient-dense foods such as fruits, vegetables, whole grains, lean proteins, and healthy fats is key to providing the body with essential vitamins, minerals, and antioxidants. These foods support various bodily functions, including metabolism, immunity, and cognitive function, while also reducing the risk of chronic diseases such as heart disease, diabetes, and certain cancers.

2. Portion Control: Practicing portion control helps prevent overeating and promotes mindful eating habits. By being mindful of portion sizes and listening to hunger cues, individuals can better regulate calorie intake and maintain a healthy weight. Portion control also allows for greater flexibility in food choices, as no foods are off-limits when consumed in moderation.

3. Hydration: Staying hydrated is vital for overall health and well-being. Drinking an adequate amount of water throughout the day helps regulate body temperature, support digestion, flush out toxins, and maintain proper hydration levels. Opting for water or other low-calorie beverages over sugary drinks can also help reduce calorie intake and support weight management.

4. Physical Activity: Incorporating regular physical activity into daily routines is essential for maintaining cardiovascular health, muscle strength, and flexibility. Engaging in activities such as walking, jogging, cycling, swimming, or strength training not only improves physical fitness but also enhances mood, reduces stress, and promotes overall well-being.

5. Mindful Eating: Practicing mindful eating involves paying attention to hunger and fullness cues, savoring each bite, and being present during meals. By slowing down and fully experiencing the sensory aspects of eating, individuals can cultivate a healthier relationship with food, prevent overeating, and improve digestion.

6. Self-Care Practices: Prioritizing self-care practices such as adequate sleep, stress management, and relaxation techniques is essential for overall health and well-being. Getting enough sleep allows the body to rest and repair, while stress management techniques such as meditation, yoga, or deep breathing promote relaxation and reduce the risk of chronic stress-related health issues.

Choosing healthy options encompasses various aspects of lifestyle choices, including nutrition, physical activity, hydration, mindful eating, and self-care practices. By prioritizing nutritious foods, portion control, hydration, regular physical activity, mindful eating, and self-care practices, individuals can optimize their health and well-being, reduce the risk of chronic diseases, and enjoy a higher quality of life. Making informed and conscious decisions about lifestyle habits is essential for achieving long-term health goals and promoting overall wellness.

Portion Control Techniques

Portion control techniques are fundamental for maintaining a balanced diet and managing weight effectively. By understanding portion sizes and implementing strategies to control portions, individuals can better regulate calorie intake, prevent overeating, and promote overall health. Here's a comprehensive look at various portion control techniques and their importance:

1. Use Visual Cues: Visual cues such as hand sizes, household objects, or food packaging can help estimate appropriate portion sizes. For example, a serving of meat should be about the size of a deck of cards, a serving of grains should be about the size of a tennis ball, and a serving of cheese should be about the size of a pair of dice.

2. Measure Portions: Using measuring cups, spoons, or a kitchen scale to portion out food can provide a more accurate assessment of serving sizes. Measuring ingredients before cooking or serving can help prevent overestimating or underestimating portion sizes and ensure that meals are balanced and nutritious.

3. Divide Plate Proportions: Dividing the plate into sections can help control portion sizes and create a balanced meal. Aim to fill half the plate with non-starchy vegetables, one-quarter with lean protein, and one-quarter with whole grains or starchy vegetables. This method ensures that meals are nutrient-dense and contain appropriate portions of each food group.

4. Practice Mindful Eating: Mindful eating involves paying attention to hunger and fullness cues, savoring each bite, and being present during meals. By slowing down and fully experiencing the sensory aspects of eating, individuals can better recognize when they are satisfied and avoid overeating.

5. Use Smaller Plates and Bowls: Using smaller plates and bowls can trick the brain into thinking that portions are larger than they actually are. This can help reduce the tendency to overeat and promote portion control without feeling deprived.

6. Pre-Portion Snacks: Pre-portioning snacks into individual servings can help prevent mindless eating and control calorie intake. Dividing snacks such as nuts, trail mix, or chips into small bags or containers makes it easier to grab a single serving and avoids eating directly from the package, which can lead to overconsumption.

7. Listen to Hunger Cues: Pay attention to hunger and fullness cues, and eat only when hungry and stop when satisfied. Avoid eating out of boredom, stress, or emotional reasons, and practice mindful eating to foster a healthier relationship with food.

Portion control techniques are essential for maintaining a balanced diet, managing weight, and promoting overall health. By using visual cues, measuring portions, dividing plate proportions, practicing mindful eating, using smaller plates and bowls, pre-portioning snacks, and listening to hunger cues, individuals can better regulate calorie intake, prevent overeating, and enjoy a healthier relationship with food. Incorporating these portion control techniques into daily routines can contribute to long-term success in achieving health and wellness goals.

Managing Alcohol Consumption

Managing alcohol consumption is crucial for maintaining overall health and well-being, as excessive alcohol intake can have a range of negative effects on physical, mental, and emotional health. By understanding the risks associated with alcohol and implementing strategies to moderate consumption, individuals can enjoy the occasional drink while minimizing harm. Here's a comprehensive look at various aspects of managing alcohol consumption and its importance:

1. Know Your Limits: Understanding recommended guidelines for alcohol consumption is essential for managing intake. In many countries, moderate drinking is defined as up to one standard drink per day for women and up to two standard drinks per day for men. It's important to be aware of these guidelines and stay within recommended limits to minimize health risks.

2. Monitor Serving Sizes: Be mindful of serving sizes when consuming alcohol, as portion sizes can vary widely. A standard drink typically contains around 14 grams of pure alcohol, which is equivalent to 12 ounces of beer, 5 ounces of wine, or 1.5 ounces of distilled spirits. Knowing how much alcohol is in each serving can help prevent overconsumption.

3. Stay Hydrated: Alternate alcoholic drinks with water or other non-alcoholic beverages to stay hydrated and pace yourself. Drinking water between alcoholic beverages can help slow down alcohol absorption, reduce the risk of dehydration, and prevent excessive drinking.

4. Eat Before Drinking: Consuming a meal or snack before drinking alcohol can help slow down the absorption of alcohol into the bloodstream and reduce its effects on the body. Eating foods that are high in protein, fiber, and healthy fats can help stabilize blood sugar levels and minimize alcohol's impact.

5. Set Limits and Stick to Them: Establish personal limits for alcohol consumption and stick to them. Be mindful of social pressures to drink more than you're comfortable with and politely decline additional drinks if you've reached your limit. Setting boundaries and knowing when to say no is essential for maintaining control over alcohol consumption.

6. Avoid Binge Drinking: Binge drinking, defined as consuming a large amount of alcohol in a short period, can have serious health consequences and increase the risk of alcohol-related accidents, injuries, and long-term health problems. Avoid binge drinking by pacing yourself, knowing your limits, and practicing moderation.

7. Seek Support if Needed: If you find it difficult to control your alcohol consumption or if drinking is negatively impacting your life, seek support from friends, family, or a healthcare professional. There are many resources available for those struggling with alcohol misuse, including support groups, counseling, and treatment programs.

Managing alcohol consumption is essential for promoting overall health and well-being. By knowing your limits, monitoring serving sizes, staying hydrated, eating before drinking, setting boundaries, avoiding binge drinking, and seeking support if needed, individuals can enjoy alcohol responsibly while minimizing harm. Practicing moderation and making informed choices about alcohol consumption can help maintain a healthy balance and reduce the risk of alcohol-related health problems in the long term.

Conclusion

Maintaining a Healthy Lifestyle

Maintaining a healthy lifestyle is essential for promoting overall well-being and reducing the risk of chronic diseases. It involves making informed choices about nutrition, physical activity, sleep, stress management, and self-care practices. Here's a comprehensive look at various aspects of maintaining a healthy lifestyle and their importance:

1. Nutrition: Eating a balanced diet rich in fruits, vegetables, whole grains, lean proteins, and healthy fats provides essential nutrients that support overall health and vitality. By prioritizing nutrient-dense foods and limiting processed and sugary foods, individuals can fuel their bodies with the nutrients they need to thrive.

2. Physical Activity: Regular exercise is crucial for maintaining physical fitness, managing weight, and reducing the risk of chronic diseases such as heart disease, diabetes, and certain cancers. Aim for at least 150 minutes of moderate-intensity aerobic activity or 75 minutes of vigorous-intensity aerobic activity per week, along with muscle-strengthening activities on two or more days per week.

3. Sleep: Getting an adequate amount of quality sleep is essential for overall health and well-being. Aim for 7-9 hours of sleep per night and establish a consistent sleep schedule to support healthy sleep patterns. Adequate sleep promotes cognitive function, mood regulation, immune function, and physical recovery.

4. Stress Management: Chronic stress can have a negative impact on physical and mental health, leading to a range of health issues such as high blood pressure, weakened immune function, and mood disorders. Practicing stress management techniques such as meditation, deep breathing, yoga, and mindfulness can help reduce stress levels and promote relaxation.

5. Hydration: Staying hydrated is essential for maintaining proper hydration levels, supporting digestion, regulating body temperature, and promoting overall health. Aim to drink plenty of water throughout the day and limit sugary drinks and alcohol, which can contribute to dehydration.

6. Social Connections: Building and maintaining social connections is important for mental and emotional well-being. Surrounding oneself with supportive relationships, engaging in social activities, and fostering meaningful connections with others can help reduce feelings of loneliness and promote a sense of belonging and community.

7. Self-Care Practices: Prioritizing self-care practices such as relaxation, hobbies, and leisure activities is essential for reducing stress, promoting self-esteem, and enhancing overall quality of life. Taking time for oneself to rest, recharge, and engage in activities that bring joy and fulfillment is crucial for maintaining a healthy work-life balance.

Maintaining a healthy lifestyle involves making informed choices about nutrition, physical activity, sleep, stress management, social connections, and self-care practices. By prioritizing these aspects of health and well-being, individuals can optimize their physical, mental, and emotional health and enjoy a higher quality of life. Incorporating healthy habits into daily routines and seeking balance in all aspects of life is key to achieving long-term health and vitality.

Enjoying Delicious and Nutritious Meals

Enjoying delicious and nutritious meals is essential for promoting overall health and well-being while satisfying the palate and nourishing the body. By incorporating a variety of nutrient-rich ingredients and flavorful spices, individuals can create meals that are both satisfying and beneficial to their health. Here's a comprehensive look at various aspects of enjoying delicious and nutritious meals and their importance:

1. Variety of Nutrient-Rich Foods: Incorporating a variety of nutrient-rich foods into meals ensures that the body receives essential vitamins, minerals, antioxidants, and macronutrients needed for optimal health. Include a colorful array of fruits, vegetables, whole grains, lean proteins, and healthy fats to provide a diverse range of nutrients and flavors.

2. Balanced Macronutrients: Building meals with a balance of carbohydrates, proteins, and fats helps stabilize blood sugar levels, support energy levels, and promote satiety. Aim to include a source of protein, such as lean meats, poultry, fish, tofu, beans, or legumes, along with complex carbohydrates and healthy fats in each meal.

3. Flavorful Spices and Herbs: Adding flavorful spices and herbs to meals enhances taste and aroma without the need for excessive salt, sugar, or unhealthy fats. Experiment with a variety of herbs and spices such as garlic, ginger, turmeric, cumin, paprika, basil, cilantro, and rosemary to elevate the flavor profile of dishes.

4. Mindful Eating: Practicing mindful eating involves savoring each bite, paying attention to hunger and fullness cues, and being present during meals. By slowing down and fully experiencing the sensory aspects of eating, individuals can enhance their enjoyment of food and cultivate a healthier relationship with eating.

5. Home Cooking: Cooking meals at home allows individuals to have greater control over ingredients and portion sizes, making it easier to create nutritious and delicious dishes. Experimenting with different cooking methods and recipes can spark creativity in the kitchen and inspire a love for cooking and culinary exploration.

6. Social Dining: Sharing meals with family and friends fosters social connections and enhances the dining experience. Whether it's hosting a dinner party, dining out at a restaurant, or enjoying a picnic in the park, sharing delicious and nutritious meals with loved ones creates lasting memories and strengthens relationships.

7. Seasonal and Local Produce: Incorporating seasonal and locally sourced produce into meals ensures freshness, flavor, and nutritional value. Seasonal fruits and vegetables are at their peak ripeness and offer optimal taste and nutritional benefits, while supporting local farmers and reducing environmental impact.

Enjoying delicious and nutritious meals involves incorporating a variety of nutrient-rich foods, balancing macronutrients, using flavorful spices and herbs, practicing mindful eating, cooking at home, dining socially, and choosing seasonal and local produce. By prioritizing these aspects of meal enjoyment, individuals can nourish their bodies, delight their taste buds, and promote overall health and well-being. Embracing the pleasure of eating nutritious and flavorful meals fosters a positive relationship with food and supports a lifelong commitment to healthy eating habits.

Made in the USA
Monee, IL
12 May 2024

58373217R00079